1994

Homeless Children: The Watchers and the Waiters

THE CHILD & YOUTH SERVICES SERIES:

EDITOR-IN-CHIEF

JEROME BEKER, *Director and Professor, Center for Youth Development and Research, University of Minnesota*

Homeless Children: The Watchers and the Waiters

Nancy A. Boxill, PhD
Editor

The Haworth Press
New York • London

Homeless Children: The Watchers and the Waiters has also been published as *Child & Youth Services*, Volume 14, Number 1 1990.

The Haworth Press, Inc., 10 Alice Street, Binghamton, NY 13904-1580
EUROSPAN/Haworth, 3 Henrietta Street, London WC2E 8LU England

Library of Congress Cataloging-in-Publication Data

Homeless children: The watchers and the waiters / Nancy A. Boxill, editor.
    p. cm.
    "Has also been published as Child & youth services, volume 14, number 1, 1990" – T.p. verso.
    Includes bibliographical references and index.
    ISBN 0-86656-789-5
    1. Homeless children – United States. I. Boxill, Nancy A.
HV4505.W27   1990
362.7'08'6942 – dc20

                                         90-30434
                                          CIP

Homeless Children:
The Watchers and the Waiters

CONTENTS

ABOUT THE EDITOR

Nancy A. Boxill, PhD, is the Fulton County Commissioner for District 6. Dr. Boxill operates three shelters for homeless women and children in Atlanta, Georgia, serving as Program Specialist for the Young Women's Christian Association. Dr. Boxill received her undergraduate degree in psychology from Duquesne University in Pittsburgh, Pennsylvania, her master's degree in psychology from the New School for Social Research in New York City, and her doctorate in child psychology from Union Graduate School in Cincinnati, Ohio.

Acknowledgement

There are many colleagues, friends and family without whom this project would never have been completed. I thank you all. For the wonderful openness and precious special moments I have shared with many children in Atlanta shelters, I am enriched. Perhaps this volume will shorten the time you spend watching and waiting.

Nancy A. Boxill

Introduction

Nancy A. Boxill

I know of a small boy eight years old who sat alone on a park bench five or six hours every day for almost a week. He alternately played with the pigeons, watched the passing people, made patterns in the air with his feet and legs or looked blankly into space. On the fourth day of his visit to this bench a friend of mine asked this boy why he sat there every day. He replied that his mother brought him there in the mornings telling him to wait there while she looked for a job and a place for them to stay. There was no place else for him to go. When asked what he did all day he simply said that he watched and he waited. He watched the pigeons and the people. He made a game of guessing where each had to go. He said that mostly he just waited for his mother to come at the end of the day so they could wait together until the night shelter opened. This volume explores and describes aspects of the life of this child and the legions of other homeless children. They are the watchers and the waiters who only now are receiving our attention.

A requisite search of the popular and professional literature reveals that while there is considerable material available about "homelessness" there is very little material available about homeless children. Although all data shows that children and families are the fastest growing segment of the homeless population, few researchers have focused attention on this population. There are perhaps a dozen researchers who travel the lecture and conference circuit. Although we enjoy each other's company and are stimulated by the collegial discourse, we regret the lack of attention that homeless children have received.

By definition then this volume is unique, timely and on the cutting edge of the research, policy and practice arenas. It is unique because it represents an interdisciplinary approach to understanding the children and the issues. It is timely in its release as a single source of research, policy and practice data. The professional discourse contained herein represents the cutting edge of thought on both the issue of homeless children and the resolution of the problem. Each author has been careful to conclude his/her presentation of data with a section on policy and/or practice implications. The volume is organized to present a logical and contextual sequence of new information, new understandings and new directions.

The first chapter sets the tone for the volume. It creates a context for understanding the circumstance of homelessness and the impact of homelessness on children. Dr. Rivlin, an environmental psychologist, takes the reader beyond the pedantic question of impact, into a discussion of the meaning of personal space and personal place in the lives of children. Through Rivlin's discussion of attributed meanings to space, place, affiliations, connections and relationships, the reader is challenged to reformulate the question of impact and effect of homelessness on children. Rivlin's commitment to understanding the emotional and circumstantial context for a child's behavior is extremely valuable. It is in the first chapter that the reader begins to reframe his/her concept of the relationships we know to be crucial for a child's growth into a healthy adult. Understanding the salient concept of home as a personal descriptor may alter measurably the reader's thought and professional practice.

In the second chapter Ellen Bassuk and Ellen Gallagher begin the documentation of the specific psychological effects of shelter-living on the behavior patterns of childhood. Bassuk and her co-authors are widely cited in studies of homeless children. Many consider her work to be the pivotal work from which all other departs or descends. Bassuk was criticized for uncovering, perhaps even highlighting, psychopathology among homeless children in her early work. Bassuk and Gallagher discuss the results of psychological measures and assessments conducted on homeless children in Massachusetts. The chapter includes the presentation of quantitative, qualitative data. Attention is focused on apparent developmental delays, observed coping, adaptive and aggressive behavior patterns. Bassuk's early work was thought to be controversial by some and denounced by others.

In the third chapter by Hall and Maza, the experiences of those children who are "on the move," homeless but not yet living in shelters are described. The authors report the results of an eight city study conducted jointly by Travelers Aid International and the Child Welfare League of America. The children described in this study live in cars, bus stations and a host of other daily changing circumstances actively seeking stability. The chapter is particularly helpful to social workers who are often on the front-line of intervention programs. Through vignettes and clinical observations the practicing professional is provided with a foothold for understanding behavior. Classroom teachers, day care teachers and shelter providers will also find the discussion of the often anxious, awkward and developmentally delayed behaviors of these children of value in program design and implementation.

The fourth chapter by Boxill and Beaty invites the reader to construct a new context for understanding mother/child relationships among homeless women and their children. In this study, the peculiar circumstance of living in public night shelters is said to produce "out-of-order" rather than "disordered" behaviors. The circumstance of living in a public night shelter is shown by Boxill and Beaty to create a context for the weakening of mother/child relationships and family bonds. It is with literal surprise that they uncover the many ways in which shelter-living, volunteer and professional intervention actually distorts the roles and goals of the homeless child. Unlike other studies in this volume, their article captures the strengths as well as vulnerabilities, the wholeness and the disparateness of the children. The authors have used a combination of participant observation and phenomenological inquiry to produce a set of conclusions sure to be helpful to human service providers and policy makers alike.

The fifth article by James Wright leaves behind the psycho-social dimension of homelessness moving us to a discussion of the physical health status and indices of homeless children. The chapter reports the results of a study of the physical health of the population funded by the Robert-Wood Johnson Foundation. The health status and forecast for these children has tremendous implications for many areas of human services. There are economic and program implications to be drawn. This chapter perhaps more than any other points the reader toward specific points of intervention to curb contagious disease and improve the physical well-being of the subject children and all with whom they interact.

The next two chapters by Rosenman, Stein and Battle respectively focus the reader on concrete program and policy options. Rosenmann and Stein, using Washington, D.C. as an exemplar describe the horrendous difficulties and gaps created by underfunded, uncoordinated and politically unpopular programs for homeless children. The authors underscore the need for a national policy to bring to focus the good intentions, high levels of commitment and professional skills available. Without such a national policy the authors warn that not only will we fail our children, we will leave the problem unsolved. This more than any other chapter is a call for national attention and action. The article by Stan Battle provides an interesting dialogue with the Rosenman, Stein article. Battle provides a historical tracing of social welfare policy from Elizabethan Poor Laws through the New Deal, the War on Poverty and up to Reaganomics. His observations about social welfare policy as a manifestation of national values raise several questions for the reader. My own question is what is the role of the professional as advocate?

The final chapter is authored by Mark Connolly of Child Hope. Connolly masterfully discloses the life style of South America's street children. The first response of the reader is likely to be astonishment at the intricacy of such a circumscribed society. The story is absolutely moving. The second response of the reader is likely to be can this happen here? The article raises a powerful and critical question. For all of the wealth, technology and sophistication of the United States, how different are we from Third World countries that Connolly describes? How long will it take for our homeless children to create societies which are mirror images of those known to Connolly? If situations described by Connolly were superimposed upon our own circumstance, the resulting image might suggest a portrait of Dorian Gray. Too awful to gaze upon, too costly to repair.

The reader's journey may not be joyful. It will be a journey which provides much to ponder at each stop. From philosophical contexts to stark facts, there is much to consider. What shall be our response?

Home and Homelessness in the Lives of Children

Leanne G. Rivlin, PhD

ABSTRACT. An analysis of the impacts of diverse forms of homelessness in children is presented and the specific roles that homes play in people's lives. The significance of settings to social, emotional and cognitive development of children is outlined. The roles of personal space and personal places are considered including territoriality and place identity. A conception of person/place attachments is offered based on the role of lifestyle, home and neighborhood attributes, affiliations with others and the temporal patterns of these relationships. Implications for homeless children are addressed.

The article in *The New York Times* is titled "Little Street Arabs," and the writer, acknowledging "that there are no exact statistics of the number of this class" explains that:

It appears that the different homeless and vagrant children who were lodged in the various lodging houses of the (Children's Aid) Society during the past year amounted to over 10,000. . . . If we consider, in addition, the number cared for by other institutions, the number who were entirely uncared for and the number arrested by the police, we may easily believe that 20,000 is not an excessive estimate of the annual street wandering children of this city. (p. 4)

Leanne G. Rivlin is Professor in the Environmental Psychology Program, City University of New York Graduate School. Co-author of *Institutional Settings in Children's Lives* and *An Introduction to Environmental Psychology*, she currently is working on a co-authored book on public open spaces and an analysis of homelessness, each drawing on historical documentation and original research.

5

The date of this piece is February 18, 1868, attesting to the long history of homelessness for children.

In the 1860s they were called "street waifs," "street Arabs," "street children," and were treated with a mixture of pity, moral indignation and disgust. Describing them as "half-clad, ragged, vagrant, hungry-looking children, peddling or street-sweeping or pitching pennies or selling papers or blackening boots" ("Street Waifs," July 20, 1869, p. 2), the journalists listed the private charities available for these street-wandering children, among them lodging-houses that not only provided shelter and food but also "school instruction, moral teaching and a chance for labor and a permanent home." The goal of these facilities was to "promote economy, independence and honesty among the lads, and to make girls good servants or industrious women." The article closed with the question "Why, with all these charities is not the tide of childish misery diminished?"

This question resounds in contemporary times given the tremendous numbers of homeless children presently found on the streets, in welfare hotels and motels, in shelters, and living in their families' cars and vans. We can ask what this "childish misery" means for the children, what effects it will have on their development and their future lives.

It is as difficult today to count the numbers of homeless children as it was in the last century. When people have no stable addresses, when they can be tallied only when social services are used, any statistics must be regarded as rough estimates. We do know that children are among the largest groups within the population of homeless signaling a desperate need to look at them carefully and try to assess the impacts of the loss of homes.

WHO ARE THE HOMELESS CHILDREN?

The experience of homelessness for children is not a homogeneous one. There are many different kinds of homelessness and different kinds of people involved (Rivlin, 1986). It is useful, first, to recognize that the time dimension is a significant one. *Chronic* homelessness is often described by the "Bowery bum" stereotype, a form that may be accompanied by drug abuse and alcoholism. Although children do not seem to fit in this category, there is evidence that some are chronically homeless as well, living out their youths on the streets, usually with other children (Felsman, 1981; Jupp, 1985).

Periodic homelessness includes a number of forms. One type arises when personal or financial pressures cause people to leave their homes, with the homes available to them if they want to return. Another periodic homelessness occurs when migrant workers travel to work sites, often leaving homes behind. In some cases entire families travel to these places, with disruptions of various kinds, as Coles (1970) has described. Although one might place gypsies and nomads in this group, in fact, they carry their homes with them with families traveling along familiar routes with known resources and people. They usually have built homes in a specific place to which they regularly return.

Temporary homelessness results from unexpected crises, fires, hurricanes, earthquakes and floods, or even relocation to a new area. However, in many cases the social resources are not totally lost. Families and friends may be there to assist, unless they too have become victims. People moving to new homes may have a problem adjusting, but generally roots begin to develop in time. It should be noted that the impacts of homelessness may differ for different members of the family. In the case of relocation for a job, the employed member may adapt more rapidly than the others. While an assumption is made that children make new friends easily, there also is denial of the pain that accompanies disruption of their lives and roots.

The most devastating form of homelessness is the *total* form. It is a consequence of complete loss of housing, social supports and connections to a community. It may be a product of natural or people-created disasters, economic catastrophes or severe personal problems and is the most difficult to overcome. If families are involved, as they often are, children are impacted as well.

In most cases these forms of homelessness are visible. But there are many invisible or hidden homeless people who are living under precarious conditions, on the edge of homelessness. A family moving into a relative's small apartment may eventually become homeless when the strain of crowded conditions and shared resources creates tensions that force the guests to leave. Other invisible homeless are those able to groom themselves and blend into their contexts, something hard enough for an individual to accomplish but near to impossible for a family with young children.

While we assume that homeless children are part of homeless families, in fact, some are totally on their own. Taking an international view, the numbers of homeless children are enormous, estimated at 90 million in 1983 with increases as each year passes (Jupp, 1985). Children roam the streets of many countries, including the United States, but we read most about those in India, Africa and South and Central America.

A distinction has been made between the kinds of homeless children, based on their relationships to their families. Jupp (1985) has described "children *on* the street," "children *of* the street" and abandoned children. Children on the street constitute the largest group, over 60 percent of the total according to Felsman (1981; 1984). These are children who work on the streets as peddlers, beggars and pickpockets while maintaining contacts with their families. In some cases they are the families' main source of support and may be sent to the city to provide a livelihood for parents and siblings. Children of the streets, estimated at 30 percent of the total numbers, live independently, occasionally contacting their families. Throwaway children, perhaps 7 percent of all homeless street children, have been abandoned by their families and are totally on their own. In each of the different forms there may be a family-like relationship among a few homeless youths, but a stable family experience does not exist. While there have been many attempts to intervene with various kinds of social services, the numbers increase, challenging the conception that children and youths have a right to a stable, safe and secure home, nourishment, schooling, health care and protection. The absence of these basic necessities and life without a home have some frightening implications for the children and youth involved, consequences that must be addressed.

LOSS OF HOME

Loss of a home is a traumatic experience for anyone. For children this loss comes at a point in their lives when the absence of stable, nurturing settings is most injurious, when they are developing a sense of themselves, of their own identity, a sense of what they are capable of doing and their own self-worth. It is a time when some degree of consistency is important to these personal identity processes. Why this is so is a topic that is sorely in need of attention. There is a tendency to narrow the focus on homelessness to the present, failing to examine the long-range consequences, especially for children. To appreciate these costs it is useful to consider the role of places in people's lives.

THE SIGNIFICANCE OF SETTINGS

All experiences are grounded in places, in settings filled with people, objects, animals, vegetation, with sights, smells, sounds and tastes of blandness, sweetness, sourness, bitterness or saltiness. In considering the impacts of places the human participants generally are emphasized. Rarely do we find the physical qualities a concern although the field of environmental psychology has directed its attention to this gap. In fact, experiences are inseparable from their context. Growing up in an affluent suburb in contrast to an urban slum or a high-rise, luxury building as compared with a rural farm mark each experience for a child in an individual way. It may be easier to consider these contrasts when we read about extreme cases, the street children of India or South America rather than the homeless in the United States. But the settings contribute to the lifeworld of the children in each case providing different lives, different resources, different kinds of stimulation and different learning experiences.

From the time of birth, and possibly before, children's surroundings begin to shape their lives, their personalities, their cognitive, social and emotional development. Without denying the central significance of nurturing persons who surround a child, these interpersonal experiences themselves have a context, occur in different kinds of places. In the early process of separating the self from the world, in distinguishing self from others, the qualities of the surroundings, the personal and cultural attributes of the people who shape the settings all help to define the world. Two components of this process are important to describe: the development of a sense of *personal space* and the development of *personal places*.

Personal space is a term that is used to describe the "small protective sphere or bubble that an organism maintains between itself and others'' (Hall, 1966, p. 119). This bubble, which is shaped by the early experiences and the culture, remains a part of the person, forever, defining the comfort zone of close and distant contacts. It is easy to acknowledge the importance of these spaces for adults — most people are quite aware of situations where their personal space is invaded, when someone has approached them coming too close. However, it may not be so clear that these standards or norms are developed at an early age. While adults feel free to approach young children very closely, the "appropriate" distance for adults is learned gradually over time. From experiences within the intimate zone that forms the personal space emerges the most detailed sense of the world as children touch, taste, hear and smell objects and sounds that surround them. Stimulation within this zone is essential to development. While stimulus deprivation can seriously damage the child (see, for example, Provence & Lipton, 1962) there also is evidence that too much stimulation, for example, the kind that results from crowded conditions also can impair the intellectual development and health of children (Saegert, 1981). Thus, in the early years of development, two important space-related attributes develop — the discrimination of the degree to which the physical proximity of others is comfortable, and discrimination of the degree to which the stimulation of the surrounding either can be filtered out or becomes aversive, qualities important when considering the lives of homeless children.

Another attribute of personal space relates to the ability to control inputs from the outside world: the ability to withdraw either physically, by oneself or with others; or psychologically, that is, to develop strategies to cognitively leave an aversive situation (Westin, 1967). This need is no less important for children than for adults. Interviews with children and young people ranging in ages from kindergarten through high school (Laufer & Wolfe, 1973, 1977; Wolfe, 1978) revealed a developmental sequence both in conceptions of privacy and ways of obtaining it. Beginning with the recognition of the privacy rights of adults, especially that of parents, children's understanding of privacy becomes increasingly articulated and complex. What is especially impressive is children's recognition that it is important for them to have privacy at times, the expression of a need that can be identified clearly in children as early as first grade (Rivlin & Wolfe, 1985).

One way of obtaining privacy is to go off to personal places where interference from the outside ceases. Observations and interviews with children in psychiatric hospitals, open education schools and day care settings have documented the significance of privacy for children, the value of a place to retreat from the stimulation, intensity and the surveillance of institutional life (Rivlin & Wolfe, 1985). The need for a "stimulus shelter" (Wachs, 1973) has been recognized for children. When we examine the lives of children living under crowded conditions, whether in apartments filled with others, in shelters accommodating hundreds or thousands, or in a single room in a welfare hotel or motel, one can wonder how much opportunity for control over stimulation or control over space exists. Living under these conditions, often in areas where the surrounding streets are at the very least unfamiliar and often dangerous, there is little escape from the intensity, few spatial ways of obtaining privacy. The ability to control space has broad implications for children's lives, providing the basis for understanding their roles in the world and their own personal qualities and competence. This can be seen in an assessment of the functions of personal places in children's lives.

Personal places are areas that are recognized as belonging to a person, places that have come to be identified with a particular individual. In the case of adults this control over space is possible by virtue of their roles and power—the father's or mother's chair, grandmother's spot on the couch, the parent's room, the teacher's desk. For children, the appropriation of space is more difficult although the functions are much the same as for adults. This process of defining places as one's own is sometimes called *territoriality* but this term, borrowed from ethology, biology, ornithology and animal psychology has some serious limitations. While territoriality is instinctive in animals, it is optional in human beings (Roos, 1968). It may be useful as a metaphor for a range of human space-related behaviors, but it is critical to recognize that much of what is identified as a territory involves private property. Territoriality in people encompasses complex social behaviors and is tied to their social and cultural experiences (Ittelson, Proshansky, Rivlin &

Winkel, 1974). Nonetheless, it is a useful concept to apply to behavior in Western cultures since it explains why the possession and control of personal places are so important over the life span.

For children, establishing proprietary interests over places at home is one means of obtaining a sense of security, a way of mastering the stimulation, expectations, and other social and intellectual demands of the outside world. At the same time it contributes to the identity of the child. Whether it is the day care center child retreating to her cubby for a "time out," a third grade boy going to his classroom cubby during a moment of stress, a student claiming possession of the reading corner, or a child chasing her younger sibling from a play area in the foyer of their apartment, all of these reflect the value that personal places can offer. These places may be enhanced by personalization—by defining the space with markers that signal that it belongs to a particular person—signs with the name of the child, mementos, toys or other objects that provide an identity for an area and for the person who occupies it. But it must be possible to lay out these markers with some assurance that they will remain. In the welfare hotel or shelter there is little room to appropriate, other than a bed. These anonymous settings provide few opportunities for personalization, placing children and their families in an anonymous mass of other people in similar states. Possession of places and control over them in these places becomes a source of conflict rather than the quality of a home.

Personalization of spaces and the development of personal places provide children and adolescents with tangible signs that they are unique, different from others. They are one of the contributions toward place identity (Proshansky, Fabian & Kaminoff, 1983), that "substructure" of self-identity consisting of "cognitions about the physical world in which the individual lives" (p. 59). Fried (1963) has called a similar process "spatial identity" to identify this environmental contribution to the self. Proshansky and Fabian (1987) stress that place identity "should not be thought of as a stable and integrated cognitive structure" (p. 23). While there are stable aspects, there are changes "in response to properties of the physical environment" (p. 25).

We can uncover some of the dimensions of this identity by asking people to talk about environments that have been important to them over the course of their lives, including their childhood places. This process of constructing an environmental autobiography (see, for example Cooper-Marcus, 1978a, 1978b; Horwitz & Klein, 1978) has been used to sensitize architects and designers to the influence of their personal histories on their preferences for particular designs. This work emphasizes the powerful and enduring impacts that environmental experiences have on people, raising questions concerning the kinds of contributions shelters, welfare hotels and the streets will make to homeless children's identities. Certainly, these are not stable settings in the lives of individuals and families nor ones that can lay down positive images of the people residing there.

ATTACHMENT TO PLACE

One dimension of this identification with places is the degree to which people develop bonds to places that provide a sense of stability, a sense of caring and concern for the settings they occupy. Some years ago, Firey (1945) described the feelings that people have for Boston landmarks, sentiments that suggest emotional connections to particular places. In my own research on neighborhoods and public spaces (Rivlin, 1982; 1987), I have heard people describe the feeling of comfort, security, safety and "at-homeness" that places afford, leading to strong bonds that develop over time. This attachment process requires a degree of stability both in people's lives and in the setting itself, although we know that people can develop strong bonds to distant or even unknown settings. Stokols and Shumaker (1981) have distinguished between "geographical place-dependence" and "generic place-dependence": geographical place dependence involves specific places with which people are associated; in the generic form people are "dependent on a category of functionally-similar places" (p. 481). This conceptualization underlines the continuing power of places in people's lives; the power, for example, of a family's home town long left behind or a category of sacred places, churches, cathedrals, mosques, or Mecca; some of them places that may never be visited.

For most people, attachments serve direct functions, anchoring their lives and rationalizing the stimulation, heterogeneity or unpredictability that exists in the world. Without romanticizing their functions, roots or attachments serve to define the world and prevent alienation. While many have questioned the degree to which they exist in contemporary society (Sennett, 1978; Tuan, 1980), there is another voice of recognition that there are new and complex ways people are developing these connections (Lofland, 1983; Rivlin, 1987), ways that assist in stabilizing their lives, providing selective opportunities to locate meaningful social contacts and activities.

It is possible that the street children of the 1860s did have connections to places, to the neighborhoods in which they spent their days, to the missions and lodging-houses that took them in. For contemporary homeless youth, especially those placed in hotels and shelters, their existence is in limbo. In many cases the local areas are reluctant or unwilling to acknowledge that children have the right to be schooled and provided recreational, medical and social services. Often the neighborhoods in which the children are being sheltered and their last areas of residence refuse to enroll them in school, creating, at the very least, interruptions in their formal educational experiences. Schools play significant roles in children's place attachments, even when they do not provide pleasant experiences for children. When denied the stability of this significant source of social and formal learning, a serious deficiency is likely to develop.

How this occurs can be seen by examining a conception of life style and connections. I have suggested elsewhere (Rivlin, 1987) that when a neighborhood or community services a "range of needs and if these needs are concentrated within an area and are served in ways that are anchored both by time and group membership or group identity, roots to that area are likely to be deep" (p. 13). While attempts have been made to keep families together in motels, hotels and shelters, facilities for the homeless serve a narrow range of needs and do not encourage a positive sense of group identity or affiliations with other. In fact, the label of "hotel child" has emerged as the identifier for these children. It is the term used to taunt them in school and in play areas. Perhaps "shelter child" also is heard. These experiences are hardly the ingredients of place attachments. This does not deny the reality that wherever the family lives must be a temporary home. But the absence of real connections to a community, to continuous schooling, to familiar neighbors and places must be seen as a serious threat for a growing child as well as for adults.

Walking the halls of welfare hotels we can hear mothers describing the dangers inside and outside. In the large congregate shelters where families share facilities with unknown others, where beds are close together and privacy is impossible to obtain, where personal activities must take place in public, in the suburban motels far from families' former homes and familiar faces, there can be little sense of "at-homeness," little connection to communities. While there definitely is socializing, sharing and supportiveness among those in the same predicament, there also is suspiciousness, shame and distancing in order to survive. How can the basic trust that Erikson (1950) sees as the foundation of healthy development ever occur in these places?

Other articles in this volume will document the specific physical, psychological and intellectual costs of homelessness on children but it is important to recognize the circumstances that explain why the disabilities occur. It also should be pointed out that not all children show significant deficits. For many families there are sufficient personal resources, stamina or "hardiness" (Kobasa, 1982) to offset the lack of financial resources and the tremendous drain that homelessness creates. But much more needs to be known about these personal qualities and coping strategies. There are professional interests directed toward the expected pathology making it easy to ignore the qualities of survivors. A close and careful consideration of all kinds of homeless persons is needed to understand the ecology of homelessness and to delineate its impacts on children.

REFERENCES

Coles, R. (1970). *Uprooted Children The Early Life of Migrant Farmworkers*. Pittsburgh: University of Pittsburgh Press.

Cooper-Marcus, C. (1978a). Remembrance of Landscapes Past. *Landscape*, 22 (3), 34-43.

Cooper-Marcus, C. (1978b). Environmental Autobiography. *Childhood City Newsletter*, 14, 3-5.

Erikson, E.H. (1950). *Childhood and Society*. New York: Norton.

Felsman, J.K. (1981). Street Urchins of Columbia. *Natural History*, 41-48.

Felsman, J.K. (1984). Abandoned Children: A Reconsideration. *Children Today*, 13 (3), 13-18.

Firey, W. (1945). Sentiment and Symbolism as Ecological Variables. *American Sociological Review*, 10, 140-148.

Fried, M. (1963). Grieving for a Lost Home. In L.J. Duhl (Ed.), *The Urban Condition*. New York: Basic Books.

Hall, E.T. (1966). *The Hidden Dimension*. Garden City, NY: Doubleday.

Horwitz, J., & Klein, S. (1978). An Exercise In The Use Of Environmental Autobiography for the Programming and Design of a Day Care Center. *Childhood City Newsletter*, 14, 18-19.

Ittelson, W.H., Proshansky, H.M., Rivlin, L.G., & Winkel, G.H. (1974). *An Introduction to Environmental Psychology*. New York: Hold, Rinehart & Winston.

Jupp, M. (1985). From Needs to Rights: Abandoned/Street Child. *Ideas Forum*.

Kobasa, S.C. (1982). The Hardy Personality: Toward a Social Psychology of Stress and Health. In G. Sanders & J. Suls (Eds.), *Social Psychology of Health and Illness*. Hillsdale, NJ: Earlbaum.

Laufer, R.S., & Wolfe, M. (1973). *Privacy as an Age-Related Concept*. Paper presented at the meeting of the American Psychological Association, Montreal, Canada.

Laufer, R.S., & Wolfe, M. (1977). Privacy as a Concept and a Social Issue: A Multidimensional Developmental Theory. *Journal of Social Issues*, 33, 22-42.

Little Street Arabs (1986). *The New York Times*. February 18, p. 4.

Lofland, L.H. (1983). The Sociology of Communities: Research Trends and Priorities. Social Interaction. Paper presented at the meeting of the American Sociological Association, Detroit, Michigan.

Proshansky, H.M., & Fabian, A.K. (1987). The Development of Place Identity in the Child. In C.S. Weinstein & T.G. David (Eds.), *Spaces for Children: The Built Environment and Child Development*, 21-40. New York: Plenum.

Proshansky, H.M., Fabian, A.K., & Kaminoff, R. (1983). Place-Identity: Physical World Socialization of the Self. *Journal of Environmental Psychology*, 3, 57-83.

Provence, S., & Lipton, R.C. (1962). *Infants in Institutions*. New York: International Universities Press.

Rivlin, L.G. (1982). Group Membership and Place Meanings in an Urban Neighborhood. *Journal of Social Issues*, 38 (3), 75-93.

Rivlin, L.G. (1986). A New Look At The Homeless. *Social Policy*, 16 (4), 3-10.

Rivlin, L.G. (1987). Neighborhood, Personal Identity, and Group Affiliations. In I. Altman & A. Wandersman (Eds.), *Community Environments, Human Behavior and Environment: Advance in Theory and Research*. Vol 9, 1-34. New York: Plenum.

Rivlin, L.G., & Wolfe, M. (1985). *Institutional Settings in Children's Lives*. New York: Wiley.

Roos, P.D. (1968). Jurisdiction: An Ecological Concept. *Human Relations*, 21, 75-84.

Saegert, S. (1981). Environmental and Children's Mental Health: Residential Density and Low-Income Children. In A. Baum & J. Singer (Eds.), *Handbook of Psychology and Health*, Vol. 2. Hillside, NJ: Earlbaum Associates.

Sennett, R. (1978). *The Fall of Public Man*. New York: Vintage.

Stokols, D., & Shumaker, S.A. (1981). People in Places: A Transactional View of Settings. In J.H. Harvey (Ed.), *Cognition, Social Behavior, and the Environments*, 441-448. Hillsdale, NJ: Earlbaum Associates.

Street Children (1869) *The New York Times*. October 3, p.3.

Street Waifs (1869). *The New York Times*. July 20, p.2.

Tuan, Y.F. (1980). Rootedness Versus Sense of Place. *Landscape*, 24 (1), 3-8.

Wachs, T. (1973). The Measurement of Early Intellectual Functioning. In C. Meyers, R. Eyman & G. Tarjan (Eds.), *Socio-Behavioral Studies in Mental Retardation*. Washington, D.C.: American Association on Mental Deficiency.

Westin, A.F. (1967). *Privacy and Freedom*. New York: Atheneum.

Wolfe, M. (1978). Childhood and Privacy. In I. Altman & J. Wohwill (Eds.), *Children and the Environment: Human Behavior and Environment: Advances in Theory and Research*, Vol. 3, 175-222. New York: Plenum.

The Impact of Homelessness on Children

Ellen L. Bassuk, MD
Ellen M. Gallagher, MA

work the article

ABSTRACT. In the past several years, families with children have joined the ranks of the homeless in significant numbers. These families now constitute a third of the homeless population and are rapidly growing. This article describes the effects of growing up in shelters and welfare hotels, and discusses various coping strategies that children have developed to adapt to the stresses of homelessness. It includes a summary of what is known about the children's developmental, emotional and learning needs.

HOMELESS MOTHERS:
GENERAL CHARACTERISTICS

Children, particularly preschoolers, are completely dependent on their families, especially their mothers. The following description of the mothers is based on a Massachusetts study of 80 homeless families with 151 children living in two-thirds of the 21 family shelters statewide. The families were interviewed between April and July, 1985. Data from the seven non-participating shelters suggested that their guests were similar to those in the study in terms of family composition, age, marital status, number of children and length of stay. The data appears to be reasonably representative of families residing in Massachusetts family shelters with two exceptions: (1) Latinos may be underrepresented, since the shelters are generally filled to capacity and 10 to 15 families are turned away each week at the larger facilities; (2) those with substance abuse and severe mental illness are usually excluded first (Bassuk, Rubin & Lauriat, 1986).

Ellen L. Bassuk is Professor of Psychiatry at Harvard University and Executive Director of The Better Homes Foundation. Ellen M. Gallagher is Research Associate for this project.

19

Ninety-one percent of the Massachusetts sheltered families were headed by women with an average age of 27 years. Almost all were receiving Aid to Families with Dependent Children (AFDC), 60% for longer than two years. The families had moved an average of four times in the year before becoming homeless and almost 40% had been doubled up in overcrowded apartments with friends or relatives just prior to the current shelter stay. More than half had resided in shelters or welfare hotels at some time in the previous five years, suggesting that for many homelessness had become a chronic problem. Surprisingly, most mothers tended to move in the neighborhood where they grew up and to be sheltered in emergency facilities in that community (Bassuk, Rubin & Lauriat, 1986).

Researchers have described how poor women who survive in the community depend on extensive kin and non-kin domestic networks, primarily composed of other women (Stack, 1974 & Susser, 1982). Homeless women, in contrast, tend to have limited relationships. When asked to name three persons whom they could depend on during times of stress, 43% were unable to name anyone or could name only one person; almost a quarter named their minor child as a major emotional support (Bassuk, Rubin & Lauriat, 1986).

The homeless mothers tended to be born into "intact" families with father present, but by adolescence almost two-thirds were living in families headed by women. The majority of their mothers had worked and did not rely on welfare for support. However, the prevalence of family violence was high (Bassuk & Rosenberg, 1987). Many of the now homeless mothers reported that they had been abused as children by their mothers and more recently, had been abused by their husbands or boyfriends. Not surprisingly, 22% of the mothers were being actively investigated for child abuse and neglect under the Massachusetts Care and Protection Law.

HOMELESS CHILDREN

General Characteristics

The Massachusetts-sheltered homeless children ranged in age from 6 weeks to 18 years (Bassuk & Rubin, 1987). Approximately two-thirds were five years or less. The number of boys and girls were about equal. An approximately equal percentage were white and non-white.

Preschoolers: Developmental Problems

Using the Denver Developmental Screening Test, an instrument utilized by pediatricians to identify gross developmental delays, we found that almost half of the 81 preschoolers (5 years and less) tested suffered from developmental lags. Surprisingly, these deficits were not confined to only one of the four areas tested — language development, fine motor coordination, gross motor skills, and personal/social development. One third of the children manifested more than two developmental lags. The homeless preschoolers from the Boston area were in most trouble; almost three-quarters had at least one developmental delay (Bassuk & Rubin 1987).

The following case illustrates some of the developmental difficulties manifested by homeless preschoolers. Five-month-old Sarah and 16-month-old Matthew have been staying with their 26-year-old mother, Martha, in a family shelter for the past three weeks. Martha had grown up in a religious family that was tyrannically ruled by her father. He beat the children for even the most minor infraction. Despite the abuse, Martha described feeling "heartbroken" after he died when she was 14 years old.

Martha graduated high school with honors and completed three years of college when she met her husband. Six months later they were married, but he was arrested and sent to jail for stealing. Feeling abandoned and disappointed, she became depressed and was briefly hospitalized psychiatrically. After his release from prison a year later, they moved to Boston to be near his family and to try to make the marriage work. According to Martha, "things fell apart because he wanted to run the streets and be independent." The next three years were marked by frequent and chaotic separations from her husband, approximately 15 moves to friends and family members, the birth of her two children, and stays in abandoned buildings, in a welfare hotel and now in a family shelter.

Five-month-old Sarah is a frail-looking, listless child, who has moved four times since her birth. She weighs slightly under 11 pounds and is being followed closely by a family doctor because of a serious feeding problem. Mother says she "spits up and can't hold milk down." On the Denver, she lagged in all areas tested. She was unable to grasp a rattle and rarely vocalized or smiled. Her 16-month-old brother, who had moved seven times since his birth, was a shy, withdrawn, quiet child. On arrival at the shelter, he stopped saying the few words he knew, refused to eat, and had trouble sleeping. He also failed in the four major areas tested on the Denver.

Martha said that she was too embarrassed to apply for a job or look for an apartment because of her appearance. She had received no dental care for many years and her teeth were black and carious. The shelter staff were helping her apply for treatment at a nearby dental clinic.

School-Age Children

The school-aged children (6 years and older) were severely anxious and depressed. Based on the Children's Manifest Anxiety Scale, approximately a third required psychiatric referral and evaluation. Scores on the Children's Depression Inventory indicated that more than half required psychiatric evaluation (Bassuk & Rubin, 1987).

The case of Robert illustrates some of the difficulties experienced by homeless school-age children, as well as the pressures of shelter life. Robert was an overweight 12-year-old boy. He said that he hated school, was bored, and worried that schoolmates would discover he had no real home. He disliked the shelter and the other children there, and spoke wistfully of the family's last home in a trailer. On several items on the depression scale, Robert checked off the worst possible response out of three. He said that he was ugly, had often thought about killing himself and would do it if he had the chance. He was not sure how he would carry this out, but felt desperate enough to hold it as an idea. Robert then supplied proof of his all-around unacceptability. He said that he had no friends. He was teased by peers and criticized by adults. He was failing in school and had already repeated a grade. (House Comm. on Gov. Operations, 1986 p. 78)

Not surprisingly, he also scored very high on the anxiety scale.

Shelter staff reported that school attendance tended to be irregular, usually because shelters are located far away from the school and adequate transportation is lacking. Twelve-year-old Jason described "his frustration at missing five weeks of school during their move (from their Staten Island apartment to a Manhattan welfare hotel) and how he commuted from the Prince George Hotel to Staten Island to attend his regular school" (Chavez, 1987). Some mothers view their homelessness as temporary and keep their children out of school until they find permanent housing; for others, however, days and weeks without a home may rapidly turn into months and even years.

According to parents, 43% of the children had already repeated a grade, 25% were in special classes, and almost 50% were currently failing or doing below average work in school (Bassuk & Rubin, 1987). The following case illustrates a range of school difficulties experienced by homeless children. Laura is a 35-year-old woman who became seriously depressed after her husband disappeared. She is the mother of three children: 11-year-old Terry, 9-year-old Jimmy, and 8-year-old Eric. The family has been living in a shelter for the past 6 months and the children have been attending school erratically. In the past five years they have moved eight times, have also been sharing overcrowded apartments with friends and family, and have lived in several welfare hotels. All three children have serious school problems. Terry has already repeated the fourth grade once and is doing below average work in arithmetic and spelling. After Jimmy repeated the third grade, he was put in a special class; he is withdrawn and has a severe speech and memory problem. Eric is currently doing average work in school but has repeated the first grade.

HOW DO CHILDREN COPE WITH BEING HOMELESS? ADAPTIVE STRATEGIES

The Massachusetts study of homeless children does not distinguish among developmental, emotional and learning difficulties associated with a life of chronic poverty, deprivation and disruption, and those problems that result from shelter life alone. In other words, many children come to shelters for the first time already suffering from serious developmental deficits, anxiety, depression, and school difficulties. However, anecdotal accounts from shelter staff and homeless mothers suggest that, in general, the pressures of shelter living exacerbate the children's difficulties and may even create additional ones. Some children seriously regress or manifest various behaviors that are attempts to cope with the stresses of homelessness, generally, and of shelter/hotel living, specifically.

Shelter and Hotel Living

Although shelters offer refuge to many families, the stresses of shelter life are many; the quality of the sheltering facilities varies by region and type of facility. In Massachusetts, small neighborhood-based family shelters are open 24 hours a day, while in other states the families must leave after breakfast and return for dinner (Bassuk, Rubin & Lauriat, 1986 & Boxill & Beaty, 1987). In New York City, a New York State Appellate Division court has ordered that all homeless families be provided with emergency shelter: 74% are housed in welfare hotels, 11% in barrack-type shelters without private rooms, 8% in family centers where each family has its own apartment unit, and 6% in shelters that have private sleeping areas, but shared bathroom and dining facilities.

Regardless of the type of facility, however, quarters are generally cramped and families have little privacy. There is a lack of both physical and emotional space. Guests are subjected to the various stresses, problems and behavioral patterns of each family. Boxill and Beaty (1987) described how all aspects of the mother-child relationship, which were formerly private, are now ". . . conducted in full public view," a situation that contributed to the "unraveling of the mother role." The atmosphere in the shelter is generally volatile and it is not uncommon for mothers to discharge tension by arguing with each other, most often about their children's behaviors. Mealtime, in particular, is very stressful since mothers must prepare and feed their children in communal kitchen and dining areas.

Most mothers are concerned about the survival of their families, and feel overwhelmed with the tasks of providing for their children and trying to make "ends meet." Many worry about functioning effectively as single parents and are understandably anxious and depressed about being homeless. Not surprisingly, they often have little energy left to mother their children consistently. Also, because of the lack of child care, mothers spend 24 hours a day with their children and must sleep in the same room, and sometimes in the same bed, with the whole family. Homeless mothers rarely have time for themselves.

The stresses of hotel living are somewhat different, and perhaps more harmful to children. Families are often isolated from other families, and because of the lack of accessible transportation, from a network of services. "Whereas shelters offer regular contacts with other families, staff persons and various resources, such as laundry facilities, telephone, meals and transportation, hotels provide a room and little else. Families live "behind closed doors," usually without access to common areas for recreation and communication (Gallagher, 1986 p. 61). The lack of structure, routine and rules compounds an already difficult living situation; hotel managers often devalue welfare families and are unwilling to provide necessary services. Furthermore, it is not uncommon for there to be illicit drug traffic and prostitution (Gallagher, 1986).

At best, life for a homeless family is uncertain and unpredictable. Mothers are severely stressed and depleted by their experiences. They frequently have little energy left to respond to and buffer their children's stress and increased neediness. In turn, the children must muster any resources they have and, to a larger degree than usual, fend for themselves. This pattern often sets up a cycle that is harmful both to the individuals and to the mother-child interaction (Boxill & Beaty, 1987).

Regressive Behaviors

It is not unusual for homeless mothers to report that after moving into the shelter their children behave differently, generally "becoming more babyish." Regressive behavior is most commonly observed in preschoolers. Many manifest eating and sleeping difficulties and start bed wetting again. One young mother said that the longer her two children, aged two and four years, stayed in the shelter the more introverted and withdrawn they became. "They now only speak in fragments and have lost a lot of the words they used to have before they got here." Another mother reported that her son could eat by himself before they moved into the shelter, but now "he can't even hold a cup of milk without spilling it." A recent description of a NYC welfare hotel described,

> four boys shooting pool, talking as tough as any New York pool sharks. One wore just his shorts, and another's face was smeared with sweat. With the boys as old as 12, they might have seemed wise about the streets — except that two of them were sucking their thumbs. Nearby, Jessie, a gangly 11-year-old, introduced a visitor to his stuffed puppy. "His name is Snuff," he said, clutching a doll that seemed appropriate for a child half his age. (Chavez, 1987 A.B1)

When people are overwhelmed by external stress or internal conflicts, they frequently return to an earlier developmental level. Their unconscious hope is to rework and master unresolved conflicts and to obtain gratification for unmet needs. Homeless children's regressive behaviors reflect their current level of overwhelming stress as well as their need for nurturance and protection.

Aggressive/Shy, Withdrawn Behaviors

Based on our experiences and mothers' reports, after becoming homeless many children seem to change, often becoming aggressive and non-compliant or shy and withdrawn. Many mothers report that their children are angry, cry for no reason, are provocative and hard to control. Some mothers commented that as their children's behavior deteriorated, the only way they could get their attention and control their aggressive behavior was to punish them physically.

A 20-year-old mother, who is now eight-months pregnant, had to leave her parents' home because of severe overcrowding. She has been living in a family shelter with her two daughters for the past three months. Five-year-old Heather is overweight, aggressive, and "won't listen to anything I tell her. She talks fresh like the other children and says things she never used to say. If I don't hit her now, she'll never listen or she'll just get worse." Mother also said that since coming to the shelter both girls have lost their appetite and will only eat if they are at grandmother's house. In contrast to Heather, three-year-old Patty is quiet and anxious, and is often scapegoated by other children because of severe eczema and a protruding umbilical hernia. She appears frightened, cries with little provocation, and clings to mother.

These observations were also validated by the results of the Simmons Behavior Checklist, an instrument used in the Massachusetts study (Bassuk & Rubin, 1987). Mothers completed a 28-item questionnaire about the behaviors of their three-to-five year old children. Each item is scored on a five-point scale, from *never* to *always*; 11 factors are derived from the 28 items. In addition, a total behavioral score is obtained and compared to normative data. In the Massachusetts study, 55 homeless children aged three to five were tested. They scored significantly higher than the mean for a sample of normal and disturbed children. Compared to emotionally disturbed children, the homeless children scored equal to or higher than the mean on the following factor scales: sleep problems, aggression, shyness, and withdrawal.

Increased aggressiveness may be a way for homeless children to express anger at their circumstances and at their parents for being unable to protect them. At the same time, unruly, provocative and aggressive behaviors are a "cry for help," a way to get more attention from adults who are depressed and anxious, and preoccupied with issues of survival. Some children use aggressive behavior as a way of imitating their parents;

> they are doing actively what they have experienced and continue to experience passively. In play they assume adult roles in which they yell, curse, and punish as an outlet for their poorly mastered aggressive drives. It appears that they use such identification with the aggressor as part of their repetitive efforts in play to master and assimilate hurtful, threatening aspects of their relationships with their parents. . . . (Pavenstedt, 1967, pp. 135-136)

Defying adults may also help them gain acceptance from peers.

Other children feel too unsafe to trust adults or to express their feelings and needs openly, and instead become shy and withdrawn.

Some have "given up" on relationships at an early age, are distrustful of adults, feel hopeless about having their needs fulfilled, and are despairing and fearful of expressing their wishes or feelings (e.g., hostility) directly. Homeless children, who have experienced the loss of a primary caretaker (e.g., father, grandparent) are often reluctant about becoming involved in another potentially disrupted relationship.

Mothering Behaviors

Homeless children seem to be searching for adults to nurture and protect them from a dangerous, uncertain and unreliable world. Boxill and Beaty (1987) have described how ". . . no part of their day was predictable. They slept in different places and or spaces every night." For some homeless children, uncertainty about their situation was compounded by their inability to depend on their parents. "They do not have inner confidence that they will not suddenly be whacked or humiliated or deserted, or that the situation will not unexpectedly change" (Pavenstedt, 1967, p. 131). A five-year-old homeless boy who had been sexually abused asked a staff person to write the following message to his mother: "Please keep us company." "Us" referred to him and three younger brothers, aged 8 months to 3 years.

Sometimes siblings turn to each other for nurturance and protection. Thirteen-year-old Laura and Patricia have been inseparable since they became homeless two years ago. They are always together and to make up for their mother's inability to care for them, they fiercely support each other. Despite their mother's generally irresponsible behavior and the families constant moving, they have attended school regularly and have received above average grades. They are generally more functional than their mother and try both to nurture and discipline her.

The sisters' concerns about survival and protection have unfortunately been enacted literally since Laura is a brittle juvenile diabetic; she has been repeatedly hospitalized because of dangerously high blood sugar levels that resulted from mother's neglect of her medical and dietary needs. Pat has taken on the responsibility of helping to regulate her sister's diet. Three months ago Laura was rehospitalized for regulation of her diabetes. During this time, Pat noticeably regressed, began talking in a babyish manner, and missed several days of school. Although the doctors wanted to place Laura in foster care, Department of Social Services intervened to keep the family together because of the sister's interdependence. They wanted to give mother "one more chance" to attend more closely to her daughter's needs.

Another coping strategy is for children to identify with the nurturant mother and to try to replace her. Sam, a four-year-old boy, assumed the care of his three-month-old brother, David, who was born two months prematurely. He mimics his mother's maternal behaviors and at times seems to be a better and more devoted mother. His 24-year-old mother considers Sam "a responsible adult" and gave him permission to feed the baby, carry him around and baby-sit. When mother is in the shower, doing errands or making phone calls, he assumes full responsibility for both David and his two-year-old sister. One of the shelter staff commented that "he doesn't seem to be having a childhood and is instead moving directly into becoming a parent."

Sometimes, the child's identification with the nurturant parent becomes pathological. Annette, a 37-year-old black single mother of four children (ages 17 years to 6 months) and cocaine user has been homeless for 5 months. She is involved in a destructive symbiotic relationship with Susan, her 17-year-old daughter. Susan had been in various foster care placements and was sexually abused. She is overweight, very immature, and has extremely poor hygiene. Last summer Susan worked, but mother took her money to buy drugs.

Recently, mother disappeared for three days leaving the younger children in Susan's care. Susan dressed up like mother, putting on excessive makeup and flamboyant clothes, and acted out sexually. She then claimed she was pregnant. When mother returned, she insisted that Susan was infertile and that, in fact, she was pregnant and had scheduled an abortion. When mother left, Susan felt hurt and angrily talked about mother's inability to parent, and her mother's drug use and sexual involvements. When mother returned she denied any negative feelings toward her. Susan now has an option to move into a residential treatment program, viewing the opportunity favorably only while mother was away. Although mother superficially supports this move, she emotionally imprisons Susan by making her feel that no one in the family can survive without her. So far, Susan has been unable to leave and continues to function as the primary caretaker in the family.

Boxill and Beaty (1987) interpreted some of these mothering behaviors (such as those in the first two examples in this section) as indicative of the "unraveling of the mother role." They imply that these behaviors are largely contextual and result from the necessity of mothering publicly.

> Where normally it is anticipated that adults set the standards for civility, compromise, and cooperation, shelter living seemed to provoke the unraveling of that responsibility and the assumption of childlike behavior on the part of the adults. Mothers appeared to have temporarily become children along with their children.

As indicated by the Massachusetts study of sheltered homeless families, for some the disordered mother-child relationship is longstanding and pre-dates the current shelter stay. In these families, the visibility of the mother-child relationship in the shelter may be stressful, but it also provides an opportunity to help mothers parent more effectively.

PROGRAMMATIC RESPONSES TO HOMELESS CHILDREN'S NEEDS

How can we respond to the special needs of homeless families? Special programming must be creatively developed. If staff are responsive to the children's needs for structure, routine and supportive limit setting, for example, then some of the children's distress can be alleviated. Homeless children should be provided with a space in which they can engage in age appropriate behaviors — and be children again. For example, a playroom setting that is adequately staffed by shelter personnel who are knowledgeable and interested in children can serve this purpose. At the same time, it provides mothers with much needed respite from the demands of constant child care.

To respond to the children's developmental and emotional problems, a range of programs should be provided either within the shelter or in close proximity. Regardless of their location, they should ensure stable, ongoing relationships with mature adults regardless of where the family will move. These programs include infant stimulation, therapeutic day care, and head start. For example,

> head start has been the federal government's best early-childhood education and health-care program for the past 23 years. Studies have shown that Head Start children are more likely to stay out of trouble, finish high school and college and land jobs than other, similarly poor children. (*Washington Post*, 1987 p. A20)

"Despite this success, the Reagan administration has been starving the Head Start program. Funding has been increased by only 1 percent each year since 1980" (*Boston Globe*, 1986 p. 18). Unfortunately, many preschool programs for poor children have encountered similar fates.

Many homeless school-age children suffer from severe learning problems. ". . . These children go to school only sporadically; they move from school to school as they move from shelter to shelter, uprooted again and again, never part of any community" (Hechinger, 1987 p. 17). It is imperative that homeless children be identified and that special efforts be made to help them attend school. New York City school system, for example, recently offered homeless parents three options that they hoped would increase school attendance: "sending their children to the last school they attended; sending them to the last school they attended when they were in permanent housing, or sending them to schools in the same district as their temporary housing" (Roberts, 1987). Transportation and special after-school programs must also be provided. A New York City elementary school offered homeless children after-school dancing lessons, tutoring and a third meal (Daley, 1987).

Without reasonable educational opportunities, the future of homeless children will remain bleak.

CONCLUSION

Researchers have previously reported that the majority of homeless children are suffering from serious developmental, emotional, and learning problems. Our observations as well as those described in other anecdotal reports indicate that the emergency sheltering facilities exacerbate the children's existing problems and create new ones. In an effort to cope with the stresses of shelter life, mother's anxiety and depression, and profound uncertainties about tomorrow, children manifest regressive, withdrawn, and sometimes antisocial behaviors. They also assume various mothering roles. Within the context of a homeless existence, these strategies are adaptive and may help children to survive. We can only speculate, however, about the negative effects of these behaviors in other settings and about long-term effects of a homeless way of life.

It is obvious that the severity of homeless children's developmental, emotional and learning needs as well as difficulties in the mother-child interaction indicate the need for an immediate programmatic and policy response. For preschoolers, five years span critical developmental stages. Extended trauma during this time may initiate a cycle of underachievement and emotional problems that cannot readily be reversed. Similarly, for school-age children continued school failures, sometimes coupled with psychological distress, may also perpetuate a cycle of life-long difficulties. Given this profile, there is no doubt that we must respond to the plight of homeless children immediately and definitively.

REFERENCES

Bassuk, E.L., & Rosenberg, L. (1987). *Family Homelessness: Why Does it Occur?* Unpublished.

Bassuk, E.L., Rubin, L., & Lauriat, A. (1986). Characteristics of Sheltered Homeless Families. *Amer J Public Health*, 76 (9), 1097-1101.

Bassuk, E.L., & Rubin, L. (1987). Homeless Children: A Neglected Population. *Amer J. Orthopsych*, 57 (2), 279-286.

Boxill, N., & Beatty, A. (1990). Mother/Child Interaction Among Homeless

Women and Their Children in a Public Night Shelter in Atlanta, Georgia. *Child & Youth Services, 14*(1), 49-64.

Chavez, L. (1987). Welfare Hotel Children: Tomorrow's Poor. *New York Times.* July 16, B1, B5.

Daley, S. (1987). New York's Homeless Children: In the System's Clutches. *The New York Times.* February 3, B1.

Dumpson, J.R. (1987). *A Shelter Is Not A Home.* Report of the Manhattan Borough President's Task Force on Housing For Homeless Families.

Emergency Aid to Families Program (1986). Hearing Before A Subcommittee on the Committee on Government Operations, House of Representatives, Washington, D.C.: U.S. Government Printing Office.

Gallagher, E. (1986). *No Place Like Home.* A Report on the Tragedy of Homeless Children and Their Families in Massachusetts. Boston, MA. Committee for Children and Youth, Inc.

Head Start for Homeless Children. (1987). *The Washington Post.* March 28, A 20.

Hechinger, F. (1987). About Education. Plight of the Homeless. *The New York Times.* May 5.

Kronenfeld, D., Phillips, M., & Middleton-Jeter, V. (1978-1980). *The Forgotten Ones: Treatment of Single Parent Multi-Problem Families in a Residential Setting.* Washington, D.C.: U.S. Dept. Health and Human Services, Grant Number 18-P90705/03f.

Pavenstedt, E. (Ed.) (1967). *The Drifters: Children of Disorganized Lower-Class Families.* Boston: Little, Brown and Co.

Perchance to Sleep. Homeless Children Without Shelter in New York City. (1984). Coalition for the Homeless.

Roberts, S. (1987). For Homeless, Struggles Include Getting to School. *The New York Times.* April 23, B1.

Seven Thousand (7,000) Homeless Children: The Crisis Continues. The Third Report on Homeless Families with Children in Temporary Shelter. Citizen's Committee for Children of New York, Inc. October, 1984.

Stack, C.B. (1974). *All Our Kin. Strategies for Survival in a Black Community.* New York: Harper & Row.

Starving Head Start. (1986). *The Boston Globe.* 18. February 14.

Susser, I. (1982). *Norman Street: Poverty and Politics in an Urban Neighborhood.* New York: Oxford University Press.

U.S. Conference of Mayors. (1987). *A Status Report of Homeless Families in American's Cities: A 29 City Survey.* Washington, D.C.

No Fixed Address:
The Effects of Homelessness
on Families and Children

Judy A. Hall, PhD
Penelope L. Maza, PhD

ABSTRACT. This is an article about children on the move. They live with family or friends and are moving on to other friends or shelters. They may be living in vehicles, bus or train stations. Their location changes as often as daily. The article intermingles data gathered in a joint agency study conducted in eight cities with social worker observations and family vignettes. Strategies and implications for policy, public education, long and short term goals are discussed.

Travelers Aid has been associated with the homeless since the movement began back in the 1850s in St. Louis. At that time the mayor of the city became concerned about the people who were traveling west and who arrived at the Mississippi River without the necessary equipment or money to continue or complete their journey. He established Travelers Aid to provide counseling, casework services and direct assistance to homeless families and individuals. Except for the war years when the numbers increased, Travelers Aid agencies have provided services to somewhat consistent numbers and types of homeless persons.

In 1986, however, Travelers Aid agencies began reporting to their national organization that they were seeing dramatic increases

Judy A. Hall is Executive Director of Travelers Aid International, the national organization for Travelers Aid located in Washington, DC. Penelope L. Maza is Director of Research for the Child Welfare League of America in Washington, DC.

in the numbers of homeless families seeking help. Why was this happening? Who were these families? What was happening to their children? It was to answer questions such as these that led Travelers Aid International and the Child Welfare League of America to develop a joint research project. The need for the joint TA/CWLA study became apparent because the population to be studied was mobile, a transient group of people who were moving across the country and who were not necessarily living in shelters. Other studies have focused on persons living in shelters and have missed this significant segment of the homeless.

OTHER STUDIES

As early as 1970, Robert Coles described the periodic homelessness of children in families of migrant farm workers and the corresponding negative and "rootless" implications for their lives (Coles, 1970).

Other research has focused on the problems of estimating the composition and size of the homeless population. Using a variety of methods, including samples of persons spending the night in shelters as well as counting persons found in the early morning hours by searching non-dwelling places in a sample area, researchers have estimated widely differing numbers of the homeless. Estimates have ranged from 250,000 to 3 million homeless persons in the United States (Rossi et al., 1987).

Studies of families have concentrated on shelter residents and the effects of shelter life on parents and their children. Nancy Boxill and Anita Beaty (1987) studied mothers and their children living in shelters in Atlanta to look at what happens to the parent/child relationship in such a setting. The families seen by Travelers Aid were not seen in any of these studies. What then was happening to those homeless families and children "on the move?"

THE JOINT STUDY

Eight Travelers Aid agencies agreed to participate in the study: Travelers Aid Society of Detroit, Travelers Aid Society of Tampa, Community Advocates/Travelers Aid of Milwaukee, Travelers Aid

Society of Houston, Travelers Aid Society of Washington, D.C., Inc., Travelers Aid Society of San Francisco, Travelers Aid Society of Los Angeles and Travelers Aid Society of Salt Lake City. A survey form was developed jointly by the national organizations that was administered to the first 50 homeless individuals and the first 50 families seen by the agencies between October 20 and December 20, 1986. Homelessness was defined as having no place to spend the night without agency intervention.

Single adults were included to determine whether or not they had children who, although they were not with them, were affected by their homelessness. Homeless adolescents were not included unless they had a child with them or were part of a family unit. Data were collected on 404 single homeless individuals and on 163 families.

Who Are the Homeless Children?

The study looked at 340 children who were part of the 163 families. They were very young, with the average age being six years old and over half being under 5 years old. Nearly half of the children were white (46%), about one-third Black (32%), 17% Hispanic and the rest Native American or unknown. Of the school age children, 43% were not currently attending. Of those in school, 30% were behind expected grade level with those from out of the local area more likely to be behind than those who were local (45% to 30%).

> Wilburn and Violetta were not married but had lived together for the past 10 years. They had two children ages 5 and 8. When Wilburn lost his job, he decided to take the family to Detroit where he thought he could get work. They stayed in a motel while he sought employment until their funds ran out. They knew no one in the area. Their daughter had already missed 6 weeks of school. The social worker observed that she could barely read the preschool books in the waiting room.

Only one city where this study was conducted had provisions for a school at the shelter itself. In the other cities the children attended the local schools. There was frequently a delay, however, in getting enrolled. When the family was "on the move" and was planning to continue on to another city, the likelihood was that the children would not begin school at all. For those who did, the process of continually interrupting the educational process was detrimental. Thus, the children in this study were missing school and were likely to continue to miss school until the family settled somewhere. The children also reported their feelings about being "kids from the shelter" when they did attend the local school. They reported a definite stigma attached to them and expressed feelings of shame and embarrassment about being homeless.

For those children living in shelters, health care professionals believe that they are particularly at risk, physically as well as psychologically. A typical report indicated that homeless children, continually exposed to the elements, "suffer from a high incidence of upper respiratory infections, such as bronchitis or pneumonia, because they sleep in automobiles and other cold, unsuitable places" (Roberts & Henry, 1986). The workers in this study observed that 10% of the children were in obvious need of health care which likely understated the actual need. Social workers suspected that 11% of the children were either abused, neglected or both.

> The Willis family: George, his wife Anna, and their two children, Jennifer, age 5, and Kevin, age 6, arrived in Milwaukee from Lubbock, Texas. George thought that a job had been secured for him in Milwaukee by the oil company he had worked for in Texas. Because of cutbacks, the company had laid him off permanently. However, when they arrived in Wisconsin, they learned that no such arrangement had been made. No job existed. They had been living in their truck which also contained all they owned. They had been washing up at rest stops along the Interstate. Anna was very angry with George for "dragging them away from home" and the children were tense and quarrelsome. Kevin had a large bruise on his left cheek.

Other studies have focused on families and children in shelters. The most comprehensive look at children as primary victims of homelessness was conducted by Dr. Ellen Bassuk of the Harvard

University Medical School (Bassuk & Rubin, 1987). Her work in 1985 with children living in Massachusetts family shelters showed that nearly half of those studied showed evidence of one major developmental delay while one-third showed evidence of two major delays.

Where Had the Children Spent the Previous Night?

Because these families were "on the move," the children had spent the previous night in many different settings. The families' use of friends or relatives as a resource meant that 15% of the children had stayed there. Nearly one-fourth (22%) had been outside, in a vehicle, bus or train station. Another fourth (24%) had been in a shelter the previous night and were now in a new setting again without shelter. Thirteen percent had used their last funds for a motel or hotel or rooming house or other arrangement.

> Although it was very cold that day, one-year-old Becky's diaper was long overdue to be changed, and she was not wearing any shoes or socks. When the social worker asked her father about this, he said that the shoes were somewhere in the van. They had not been able to find them. Becky, her parents, and her three-month-old sister, were on their way to the West Coast where they hoped to settle. Her mother, Cindy, thought one of her uncles lived in the Salt Lake City area, but they had not been able to locate him. They were out of money, and the engine of the van was beginning to make some ominous sounds.

Homelessness was a recent experience for over half (58%) of the children, having occurred within the past month. Another fourth (235) had been homeless 1-3 months, 5% 4-6 months and 13% over 6 months. Social workers reported that the children were mirroring the attitudes of their parent(s) toward the situation. Those adults who were desperately anxious about their homeless dilemma had with them children who were also anxious, desperate, and difficult to manage. As adults became more resigned into homelessness and depressed, so were their children. The problem was worsened if the families had to be separated because shelters which could house the family together were nonexistent or filled. The implications of this mirroring phenomenon on the child's adjustment in school is certainly an area for further study.

Eight-year-old Natalie was interviewed by a reporter for a large national newspaper. "How long have you been living in the shelter?" asked the reporter. "About three weeks now," Natalie replied. "And what do you miss most from your old home?" the reporter continued. "I miss my dog . . . and it's scary here at night," the little girl sighed.

In addition to the children who were with the adults on the road, there were *77 other children* belonging to these families who were *not* with them. While half (52%) were with former spouses, the rest were scattered: with other relatives, friends, in foster care or hospitals. While not homeless, these children were, nonetheless, affected by the homelessness of their parent(s).

In addition, the individual homeless in this study were parents of *103 children*, none of which were with them. Of these children, 41% were with former spouses, 26% with relatives, 25% with current spouses and 6% were in foster care.

Loretta Johnson and her three children, ages 17, 14 and 12, arrived in Los Angeles, having moved there from New Orleans. She had been diagnosed as having lupus and diabetes, and she was separated from her husband who, she said, had a drug problem. After appealing to her family for help, Loretta was offered a place to stay with her sister and brother-in-law and their two teens who lived in a small mobile home. The inevitable occurred with the lack of space, and there was a break between the families. The 17-year-old son who had been an average student started to become difficult to manage both at school and at home. In desperation, Loretta sent him to live with another of her sisters in Baton Rouge. Meanwhile, she and the other children left her sister's after an argument. Her newly found job as a part time cook did not provide enough income for the family to move into an apartment. They had no more relatives or friends to whom to turn.

Who Were the Parents of These Children?

The female parents were on the average: 29 years old, 50% minority, and 63% unemployed more than 3 months. The male parents were on the average: 34 years old, 47% minority and 41% unemployed more than 3 months.

> Maria, a 28-year-old mother with 5 children, ages 10, 8, 6, 4 and 2 months, had fled Miami, Florida, from an abusive boyfriend. Her right eye was black behind her sunglasses, and she walked as if her body was sore. She arrived in Washington, D.C., hoping that her former husband's family would provide assistance. Her parents were deceased. This hope was dashed when the family would not even talk to her. She had been unemployed from her job as a waitress since shortly before the birth of the baby.
> Her 10-year-old son was angry, and twice the agency staff had to stop him from hitting another child in the waiting area. He was a year behind in school, and had already missed 20 days this fall as had his two sisters. The four-year old was sucking his thumb and clinging to a stuffed bear. The 8-year old kept asking when they were going to eat. This family had not eaten in 24 hours.

In over half (56%) of the families, there was only one parent (although the spouse may be somewhere else, i.e., not necessarily a single parent family). The reasons for their homelessness varied, but the underlying cause in the majority of families had to do with lack of funds due to loss of a job. The families had left their last permanent address because of loss of job (44%) or not being able to pay the rent or eviction (27%). Another reason cited was "family crisis" which may or may not have been precipitated by unemployment. About 15% stated that they wanted to visit friends or relatives or to relocate. Because these families were "on the road," it is not surprising that 80% of them were from outside the local area.

Employment

Most of the parents had been employed recently. Social workers reported a typical scenario for the two-parent families: if the mother lost her job, the family continued to be supported by the father's job. When the father lost his job, however, the family could not be supported by the mother alone. For one-parent families, single men with children became homeless sooner than did single women with children.

A study completed in 1987 in shelters in Colorado found that 76% of the mothers and 82% of the fathers had been previously employed (Colorado Children's Campaign, 1987).

The Role of Friends and Relatives

The family would typically turn to family and friends for support and shelter while they searched for employment. Over half (57%) had lived with relatives at some point in their homelessness. The longer a family was homeless, the more likely they were to have "used up" their friends and relatives. The likelihood of having lived with family or friends increased to more than three-fourths (77%) for families who had been homeless more than 3 months, as compared to 61% of the families who had been homeless 1-3 months and 47% of the families homeless than one month. Nearly half of the families which had been homeless for less than one month (43%) chose their final destination because friends or relatives were there.

The situation of being homeless and living with relatives or friends is in itself stressful. Crowding, substandard housing, leaving at the request of the landlord or other residents were all reasons why these families had left the homes of their friends or relatives. Another 10% cited "not getting along with each other" as the reason they were leaving. Since most families were seeking employment, nearly half left the homes of friends or relatives to go to a location where they thought they could find work.

Jim, Sandra and their three children under age 6 were on their way to Los Angeles from Rockford, Illinois. When Jim had lost his job, they were unable to continue to pay the rent and were evicted. They moved in with Sandra's mother who lived in a one bedroom public housing project. Sandra said that her mother, although she loved her grandchildren, became very nervous with so many little ones in such a small apartment and disapproved of the way Jim and Sandra parented them. Money was extremely tight, and the family was living on Sandra's mother's social security check which was inadequate to provide for all of them. Sandra described several heated arguments with her mother. The rules of the public housing project did not permit so many people to live in such small space, and the manager was threatening to evict the entire family. Jim hopes that he will be able to find a job in California.

The Mobile Homeless

The families in this Travelers Aid study were primarily from out of the local area (80%). They had chosen their final destination for a variety of reasons, but the two most important reasons were: jobs there (46%) and/or friends or relatives there (44%). Contrary to some common notions, only 14% indicated that one of reasons they chose a final destination was the availability of social or health services.

Families in this study came from 33 different states and 52 different counties. They were headed for 20 different states and 37 different counties. Sometimes they chose their final destination based in inadequate or incorrect assumptions about employment opportunities. For example, Travelers Aid Society of Houston found families arriving there to work in the oil industry which itself was laying off workers daily. Detroit found that families still thought there would be work in the automobile industry there. Other families were traveling long distances thinking that jobs had been promised to them, only to find that no such job existed.

Families in this study came from 33 different states and 52 different counties. They were headed for 20 different states and 37 different counties. Sometimes they chose their final destination based on inadequate or incorrect assumptions about employment opportunities. For example, Travelers Aid Society of Houston found families arriving there to work in the oil industry which itself was laying off workers daily. Detroit found that families still thought there would be work in the automobile industry there. Other families were traveling long distances thinking that jobs had been promised to them, only to find that no such job existed.

> Margaret paced the social worker's office as she alternately berated the manufacturing company which had laid her off permanently, this new city because she still could not find a job, her children for their anxiety and disruptiveness, and the social worker for not finding her a shelter that could accommodate the entire family. The shelter space available was for mothers and children under age 12. Margaret's oldest son, Kevin, age 14, would have to stay elsewhere. Margaret depended on Kevin to help with the younger three children. And besides, "Kevin will get scared over there by himself," she said. "No telling what can happen to him. . . ."

CONCLUSIONS AND RECOMMENDATIONS

Increasingly in the United States, homelessness is becoming a children's problem. The child who travels from place to place with a mobile homeless family suffers from this experience. But also the child who is left behind with or by his/her homeless parent, or by the rest of the family, suffers in a different way.

While most current research focuses on families and children in shelters, the Travelers Aid research has examined families who are mobile and not necessarily living in shelters, at least not yet. The families seen by Travelers Aid have, primarily, been employed or had a history of employment. They live from paycheck to paycheck with little or no savings. Therefore, when the plant closes or the layoff comes, and employment benefits run out, these families have no resources. They can no longer pay the rent or make the mortgage payment. When they arrive in another city, even if they can find work, they may not be able to pay the deposit on rent and utilities to enable them to get into housing.

The people that were seen by Travelers Aid were still on the move, desperately seeking new employment and new opportunities.

The TA workers reported that, to some extent, the level of desperation and anxiety of the adult family members was reflected in the children who accompanied them. As the adults became more depressed and resigned to shelter living and lack of opportunity, so did their children.

Employment

The people seen in this study who were not homeless due to relationship problems were primarily out of work. Employment is a significant issue. Each year 2-3 million Americans are permanently displaced due to changes in the work place. Some of these people are represented in the Travelers Aid sample. Secondly, even when the persons seen by Travelers Aid arrive in another city where employment opportunities exist, they may not have the necessary skills to qualify for these jobs. Training and retraining programs, as well as nationally dispersed employment information, are needed to assist displaced workers to become productive in new jobs and to stabilize their living situation.

Housing

Another extremely significant issue is the lack of affordable housing. The rising cost of housing coupled with a decrease in low-income housing assistance programs are being reflected in the numbers of homeless families. Kay Young McChesney has documented a relationship between the increased numbers of low-income families and the decrease in low-cost housing. Her study found that families become homeless because of precipitating events which center around two themes: economies and relationship crises (McChesney, 1986). This finding is documented by our TA study.

Short and Long Term Solutions

While we address these important issues at the public education, policy and legislative levels, we are witnessing a generation of children growing up without a sense of belonging anywhere. These children are victims of the homelessness of their parents and are suffering physically, emotionally, and in lagging behind in their education: the area that has traditionally held out the most promise to those caught in a cycle of poverty. Are these then the next generation of homeless, knowing no other way of life?

In the short term, we need shelters which permit families to remain intact; we need transitional housing programs where individuals and families can live while they get training or jobs and save toward the cost of moving into their own homes; we need community programs designed to assist families in the transition from homeless to stability; programs that are comprehensive in their scope to deal with the economic, the physical and the psychological components of homelessness.

REFERENCES

Bassuk, E., & Rubin, L. Homeless Children: A Neglected Population, *American Journal of Orthopsychiatry*. 57(2), April 1987: 279-286.

Boxill, N., & Beaty, A. (1990). Mother/Child Interaction Among Homeless Women and Their Children in a Public Night Shelter in Atlanta, Georgia. *Child & Youth Services*, 14(1), 49-64.

_____. Children's Campaign, Denver, Colorado: Summer 1987.

Coles, R. Uprooted Children: The Early Life of Migrant Farmworkers Pittsburgh: University of Pittsburgh Press, 1970.

_____. Homeless Coalition Survey, Pinellas County, Florida, January 1987.

_____. Homeless Families in Massachusetts: Progress and Action. (Executive Office of Human Services, January 1987).

_____. Homelessness in America's Cities (United States Conference of Mayors, June 1984).

McChesney, K. Families: The New Homeless, *Family Professional*. 1(1): 13-14, 1986.

McChesney, K. New Findings on Homeless Families, *Family Professional*. 1(2), 1986.

_____. No Room at the Inn: A Study of Homeless Families in Colorado, (Research Project conducted by Colorado).

_____. Recommendations (Ad Hoc Advisory Committee to the Division of Maternal and Child Health on the Health Needs of Homeless Children and Youth, from a meeting co-sponsored by the Division of MCH, Bureau of Health Care Delivery and Assistance, Health Resources and Services Administration, Department of Health and Human Services, and the University of Pittsburgh, Graduate School of Public Health, Department of Health Services Administration, Public Health Social Work Program, Washington, D.C., 1985).

Rivlin, L. A New Look at the Homeless, *Social Policy*, Spring 1986: 3-10.

Roberts, L., & Henry, M. (1986). State Ordered to Shelter Homeless Families. *Youth Law News* (San Francisco, July-August).

Rossi, H., Wright, J., Fisher, G., and Willis, G., The Urban Homeless: Estimating Composition and Size. *Science*. Vol. 235, 13 March 1987: 1336-1341.

————. The Growth of Hunger, Homeless and Poverty in America's Cities in 1985 (United States Conference of Mayors, January 1986).

————. Workshop on Homeless Children and Adolescents, Discussion Summary. National Institute for Mental Health Workshop, Spring 1987.

Mother/Child Interaction Among Homeless Women and Their Children in a Public Night Shelter in Atlanta, Georgia

Nancy A. Boxill, PhD
Anita L. Beaty

ABSTRACT. Public night shelters across the nation serve as a temporary resting place for hundreds of thousands of homeless families. In this article the delicate and important dyad of mother and child is described as observed in one such shelter. Through participant/observation the authors provide a look at the impact that circumstance may have on the nature and quality of mother/child interaction. Their observations provide an alternative way of understanding the experience of homeless mothers and their young children.

Virtually every major urban center in America is experiencing a growing population of homeless people. A surprisingly large number of the homeless are women and their children. This chapter does not attempt to define homelessness, estimate its proportions, report its antecedents, or suggest public solutions. Rather the focus of this study is an exploration of the relationship between mothers and their children who find themselves in a most unusual circumstance. The study begins to elucidate the experience of these families as they interact in difficult circumstances. The authors believe that until the experience of this population is carefully explored and sen-

Nancy A. Boxill is Program Specialist for Women in Crises, Y.W.C.A. of Greater Atlanta. She holds a faculty appointment at Union Graduate School and is a member of the Fulton County Board of Commissioners. Anita L. Beaty is Co-Director of the Homeless Task Force in Atlanta, Georgia.

49

sitively understood, the programs and policies designed to serve this population will succeed at best by chance. The data chosen to facilitate an understanding of the relationship of these mothers and their children is individual experience. Programs for planned change and social policy assessment must include individual experience as a data source.

Little research has been conducted on homeless women and their children. The most comprehensive study to date was conducted by Ellen Bassuk of the Harvard University Medical School. Data from this study clearly identify children as the major victims of homelessness. Bassuk reports that among preschool children one half of those studied evidenced one major developmental delay other than speech. One third of the population evidenced two major developmental delays. Among school-age children, 45% reported having repeated at least one grade in school, and most evidenced high levels of anxiety and depression (Bassuk, 1986). These are important data that provide one level of understanding. Yet there is certainly more to understand. The combination of quantitative data by Bassuk and the qualitative data of the authors increases the opportunities for the human service community to more fully understand the needs of this population.

There is little disagreement that the mother/child relationship has far-reaching and extremely important value in the healthy growth and well being of children. Documentation of the importance of this relationship is well reported by Bowlby and others in the literature on bonding and attachment. The continuing influence of the mother/child relationship on personality, self-concept and developmental foundation is well documented throughout the professional literature. There is also full realization that environment, more specifically, "personal place," is a key determinant in an individual's definition of one's self. People and places are not independent parts of living. "Personal place" describes one's group membership and potently contributes to one's definition of his/her personal qualities and abilities" (Rivlin, 1986). This study elucidates and thematizes the experience of homeless women and children who use a public night shelter and are by circumstance forced to define themselves and build their mother/child relationships in an open and public, "personal place."

SUMMARY OF DAILY EXPERIENCE

Homelessness for a woman with children means having to find a shelter that will temporarily/momentarily house her and her children. Homelessness means that mothers must always carry all of their belongings and those of their children.

Most shelters require residents to leave by 6:00 a.m. A woman with children must awaken, dress, feed her children, and repack her belongings to be sure that she and her children are ready to leave the shelter at the required hour. She must find transportation from the night shelter to a day shelter for herself and her children. The shelter opens at 7:30 a.m. but she must wait in line to be assured of securing one of only thirty available spaces for children. If she is in line early enough her children are cared for at the day shelter until 5:00 p.m. The children shelter has no space for mothers. Mothers must therefore leave their children with strangers who only temporarily visit their lives. At the end of the day, mothers must return to the shelter and begin once again the process of finding somewhere for themselves and their families to sleep.

For those mothers who cannot or choose not to leave their children at the day shelter, a long day of shouldering physical and emotional burdens begins. Some women spend their day at a women's day shelter. They tolerate the forced sharing of open public space. They simultaneously care for their children and wait for a phone call regarding a previously applied for apartment, job or social service. Other women, with children and belongings in tow, attempt to negotiate the hurdles of the employment, housing, education and health arenas.

Many of these women are young mothers who because of their youth have never clearly understood the human service or employment system nor the value each places on documents such as birth certificates and social security cards. Their lack of exposure, knowledge and sophistication hinders their success.

Most night shelters open at 7:00 p.m. Once there, the families enter through the rear door. If the mother knows that she will be late, she must call ahead and arrange to have her "space" saved until she arrives. Dinner is provided by volunteers who prepare and serve the meal at about 8:00 p.m.

Families stake claim to a space for the night. Mothers may set up a number of mats or cots for the family. Young children may fall off the cots, so a choice is often made to arrange a set of mats on the floor, in a space large enough to accommodate the whole family. Sheets and towels are provided.

Mothers take turns washing and ironing for their family, hoping that their children are occupied while they accomplish this task. If she likes, a mother can arrange a shower time for herself and her children. There are no bathtubs.

By 9:00 p.m. the children are supposed to go to bed. Many of the smaller children are asleep before this time and are the source of consternation for the older children who play on the gym floor. The older children are constantly admonished to watch out for the little ones who are trying to sleep. Some of the mothers retire to the dining area to smoke, talk, fix each other's hair, watch TV or use the telephone.

Each and every activity is done in public: that is, the women do their mothering in the company and in full view of others. We have called this "public mothering."

METHODOLOGY

Population

Forty families who used a public night shelter in Atlanta, Georgia during a six-month period comprised the population for this study.

The shelter users were not a monolithic group. The mothers ranged in age from 18 to 42. The majority were between 18 and 23 years old. Children ranged in age from 7 days to 17 years old. The group included many races, varied marital statuses and antecedents to homelessness. The only common denominator was the circumstance of being-without-a-home.

Data Collection

This study employs a qualitative methodology as a means of describing and critically analyzing the mother/child interaction among homeless women and their children who utilize a night shelter.

Qualitative methodology places the highest value on insightful understanding of human experience as the goal of social science investigation. It views human experience as the primary data for analysis. To that end, participant/observation and open-ended interviews were the selected techniques of data collection producing descriptive data which emphasizes and facilitates the understanding of a particular human experience within a specific context of social interaction (Patton, 1979). The use of these techniques permitted the researchers to participate as full partners in the experience under investigation and to express their own points of view while reporting and analyzing individual and group experiences as they unfolded. These are most desirable characteristics in social problem research (Wirth, 1979).

The open-ended or unstructured interview allowed the researchers to capture through questioning and conversation the words of the subject rather than a summary of responses. All conversational approaches were intended to elicit the subjects' understanding of their world and relationships rather than a particular piece of information or singular response. The data present the results of hours of participant observation of homeless mothers and their children.

Data Analysis

The experiences and observations reported in this article were thematized in the mode of phenomenological investigation as described by Colazzi (1975), Giorgi (1970) and Wertz (1982). The thematization of individual descriptions permits shared experiences to be grouped for enhanced understanding. It also preserves and includes peoples' own words (written or spoken), observed behavior, letters, poems, etc. (Bogden, 1975). This form of analysis benefits clinicians, program planners and policy makers. The use of quotation marks indicates the actual language used by the mothers and children.

Six themes emerged from the authors' observation. Each theme stands alone and is discussed separately in hopes that other researchers and human service professionals may be guided in important new directions for action. The overarching theme/concept which emerged was the difficulty mothers and their children as family units face in establishing and maintaining *ordered mother/child relationships* in this circumstance.

CHILDREN'S THEMES

Theme 1: Intense Desire to Demonstrate Internalized Values as a Way of Asserting Self

The hours that children spent in the night shelter were observed as essentially unstructured time. The majority of the activity was random play among children of widely divergent ages, typified by abandoned running up and down the gym. This random activity was restricted only by fixed times for meals, bathing, lights-out and early morning preparation for leaving the shelter. As a way to be non-random, or focused, many of the children observed, created ways to define, introduce, and assert themselves to each other and to the nameless volunteers who were only temporary visitors from the larger world. In their own ways the children insisted on being known from the inside. They resisted adult attempts to clump them into a category of deprived, poor or even pitiful children.

Example: Debra, an eight-year old tells me who she is on the inside as we share an experience in the kitchen of the shelter following dinner. Debra entered the kitchen and watched me begin to clean up. We greeted each other with our eyes. She asked, "Can I have a job to do?" I was pleased to include her in my work and suggested that she gather all of the serving spoons. We exchanged small talk as we worked. When she finished, she instructed me, "Give me another job." I responded immediately by asking her to cover the leftover food. Once again upon completion she said, "Nancy, can I have another job?" I asked her then to rinse out the dishcloths. When the kitchen was clean and Debra had completed her jobs she announced that she was "all done." I praised her warmly and expressed how proud I thought her mom must be to have such a good helper in the family. Debra smiled and asked, "Will you give me something for doing my jobs?" I was surprised. I prepared to give her a lecture on work and rewards. My thoughts came slowly and I simply said, "No, I have nothing to give you." Quite seriously she said, "Yes you do." My mind anticipated a request for money or more dessert. I asked, "What do I have to give?" Her eyes brightened and seemed to hide a special surprise as she said, "You can give me a hug. You can always give a hug when you have nothing else to give." Knowing Debra now from her inside and feeling embarrassed I gave her a strong, warm hug, tearful all the while. Debra had asserted herself making explicit a genuine description of her worth in the world. She provided me with a glimpse into her value system for herself and others.

Kevin, age 6, asserted his intention to be seen as a whole, choosing actor in the world. His actions in the following experience evidenced his strength in resisting a caption of "dependent urchin" gladly receiving charity. He entered the kitchen forcefully and clearly requesting more food from a group of volunteers of a local church. With pride and manners he said, "May I have seconds, but don't give me any of that chicken. I don't like it, I want the other meat." What I heard and saw was his refusal to allow nameless adults to describe his world. I watched and experienced him as feeling confident in his ability to discriminate and be known by his likes and dislikes. He was not afraid to say "no."

In so doing he readily engaged unsuspecting adults who may have had preconceived notions of him and/or his world. Kevin created a many-faceted description of himself with the use of a simple phrase.

The many ways which children of all ages continually found to state who they were astounded me. Viewed in the context of self-assertion of values and identity, in an identity-threatening circumstance, the children's "yeses" and "nos" took on new meaning. The children protected and expressed their self-esteem. (They carved out their identities and special individual capacities and qualities.) There is room for speculation on how these children came to develop their values, etc. But no conclusion can exclude their mothers as primary adults who actively embraced their roles as purveyors of values.

Mary, a 14-year old, drew a picture of a Greek goddess in 10 minutes as we talked during dinner. At her mother's prideful prompting, she listed the name and history of the goddess in the blink of an eye. Mother and child were happy, and enjoyed each other's success.

**Theme 2: Questioning the Certainty of Anything,
the Ambiguity of Everything**

For most of the children in the night shelter, "tomorrow" is a
fuzzy, ambiguous prospect. There is only the certainty of the morning routine of leaving the shelter. The remainder of the day is not
assured. Among themselves the children spoke about being different from other children they had known. Many did not go to school.
Those that did go to school feared that their peers would find out
that they had no address, no home. They had mixed feelings about
the kindness of the volunteers and strangers who brought them food
and clothes. They knew that they acquired the basic things of life in
a different way than other children.

Nothing, no part of their day was predictable. They slept in different places and or spaces every night. Among strangers, they ate
foods that were unfamiliar or prepared in unfamiliar ways. There
was no assurance that any adult would have the capacity to, or
interest in, helping them negotiate the world or bring order to daily
living. They lived in a gap of uncertainty.

For a few hours during the night their lives were influenced by
well-meaning volunteers who invited them to play games with
strange rules, encouraged them to behave in ways which exceeded
parental limits and discouraged opportunities to confront or explore
the reality of their world. The children reacted by vacillating between controlled deference, polite requests and intrusive words and
actions. They alternated between taking the ball away from a group
of volunteers and returning shortly with a request to "please play
basketball." They avoided conversations with adults, moms or volunteers, returning shortly with a verbal or physical demand for attention. They rejected the clothing brought by volunteers yet fought
over a single article of clothing selected or given to another child.
They made stealing a game yet insisted on rigid adherence to un-
compromising rules in their role as surrogate parent to younger siblings. Their behavior evidenced attempts to physically control the
volunteers by shoving, pulling or jumping on their backs.

The younger children often screamed and cried when out of their
mothers' reach. Their facial expressions bore the fear of being
abandoned. They cried over and over "mama," "mama" though
mama was within sight, not reach. It was an exaggerated response.

Many of the preschool children have retained their playfulness and hopefulness. Mary, age 5, asked Whitney, age 4 with great drama and body language, "But when will I know things? I want to know things. My mama doesn't have time to teach me (hanging her head in her hands). I don't know anything." Whitney replies, "You will know things, it just takes time. Maybe one day you can go to school." "When" is written on Mary's face. Keisha, age 9, expressed profound ambivalence about her place in the world as she hung herself around my neck asking me how many children I had. I said none; "Oh," she said, "my mom says that people who don't have children are blessed." Not believing my ears I said, "She's right, it is a blessing to have children." With firmness she said "no." She said, "people who don't have children are blessed." Her whole body asked me what I thought. I felt her question on my insides and simply hugged her, unable at that moment to assuage her uncertainty not feeling strong enough to affirm her. It was much later in the evening, before I left the shelter, that I found Keisha and told her that I was sure that meeting her was a blessing in my life.

Some of the older teens had given up on "trying to make the best of a bad situation." They sat silently, sadly and alone. Their words were "I'm o.k." but their body language said, "Please don't see me. I can't decide how I want to be seen."

Theme 3: Conflict Over the Need for Attention and the Experienced Demand for Independence

With few exceptions the children in the shelter called the female volunteers "mama" or "mommy." They reached for volunteers' hands and climbed on their backs or laps seeking physical contact. They unabashedly demanded physical attention while simultaneously disconnecting abruptly and running away. Almost in the middle of a sentence and/or game they would disappear to join a group of children playing, just as abruptly they returned to the adult.

This pattern was repeated throughout the night. They ran to their moms forcing themselves into their arms or laps then ran away to find another activity, conversation, reward or event. They seemed to want to know they could be dependent, yet needed to show that they could be independent.

Their daily life requires both. They need adults in all of the ways that children need adults. They know that they must also find ways to relieve their moms of the fear and worry that they are okay. Often in provoking fights with other children they return to tell their mom of victory or pain. Children of all ages constantly juggled the message that, on one hand, they can stick it out alone and on the other hand, mom is there for them when needed.

Theme 4: Mothers' Themes — Public Mothering

In this circumstance, among this population, mothers and their children may not ever interact in private. Every aspect and nuance of the mother/child relationship occurs and is affected by its public and often scrutinized nature. From waking to waking, mothers and their children live in shared spaces. Family units that have previously enjoyed the freedom to express love, caring, frustration, anger and all manner of other emotions in their own homes, now are forced to express their feelings in communal settings, subject themselves to prevailing shelter rules for family living, stifle their strongest and deepest feelings, expose their style of mothering" to strangers, capitulate to peer pressure and catch a glimpse of who they appear to be in the eyes of onlookers.

Yvonne, a mother of three children confessed,

> I know I sometimes do things [to my children] that somebody else expects me to do to them. I can't [even] let my seven-month old cry because he might bother the others. So one night I sat up all night in the dining room holding him . . . he was restless and whining. Other mothers had yelled at me to "get that baby quiet."

She expressed sadness and concern that her own mothering was influenced and often directed by the presence and needs of other mothers. We both wondered when and how she would carve out her own style of mothering. More importantly, we wondered how and when her children would come to really know her.

Karen, a young mother of four children was deeply sad and defeated as she talked about the stress of the daily routine of a homeless mother. "Every morning I want to cry. At five o'clock in the morning I have to wake up my children. They are not ready to wake up. They cry and get hysterical every morning. They cry for hours." Her eyes and body said, "I feel cruel, but what can I do?" The director of the day shelter commented to the authors that Karen's children and others were often very upset when they arrived.

Scenes of one mother verbally attacking another mother unfold throughout the night. Comments like, "I don't let my child do that" or "They just let their kids do whatever they want; they don't care," are voiced in accusatory tones. If one can separate the hostility and anger of the tones, the pressure of public mothering emerges clearly. When mothering is constantly unfolding in full view of the public, family life and mother/child relationships appeared to the observer and are experienced by the mother as being "out-of-order."

Theme 5: Unraveling of the Mother Role

On initial review of the data the authors believe they had observed frequent "role reversal" within families. Further, more careful review and analysis lead us to correct our terminology to more accurately reflect and report our observations and the mothers' experience. *Unraveling* was determined to be a more appropriate term. The authors regularly observed teen-aged girls taking the leadership in preparing sleeping spaces, doing laundry or caring for younger siblings. Teenagers became surrogate mothers as they disciplined, fed, bathed and bedded younger siblings. The authors came to know that such a picture was incomplete. In fact, the clear eye was able to see that mothers had not abdicated roles or responsibilities. Rather, mothers were being soothed by the efforts of their older children. In an unkind and often assaulting world, mothers were comforted by their children's special acts of assistance and caring. A nightly ritual in one family involved the combing and braiding of the mother's hair by one daughter while her other daughter carefully folded and stored the mother's clothes.

Martha, a 24-year-old mother of four children under five years of age, spoke quite clearly about the vital role her children played in her emotional well being: "I don't get depressed about not having a place to live as long as I can be with my babies. They make me happy." Similar comments from others included, "We are all we

have. It's just us alone against everybody else and that's okay."
Throughout the observations and conversations, mothers reported
that they found solace and temporary relief from emotional pain
through the role their children played in loving them. The children
were observed to have behaved and functioned by intuition or request in ways that mothers would ordinarily behave. Holding constant Erickson's concept of the mutuality of the growth process, we
believe that in this circumstance the mother's role, absent the opportunity to be provider, was "unraveling."

Instances of unraveling also included meal-time experiences.
Mothers with their children (served by volunteers) sat with petulant
faces and childish tones saying, "I don't want any squash" or
"Take that off my plate," or instructing children, "Don't eat that,
it's nasty." Mothers argued about their place in line at meal, bath,
or bed times. These incidents always occurred in the company of
children. Where normally it is anticipated that adults set the stan-
dard for civility, compromise, and cooperation, shelter living
seemed to provoke the unraveling of that responsibility and the assumption of childlike behavior on the part of the adults. Mothers
appeared to have temporarily become children along with their children.

Theme 6: The Experience of Being
Externally Controlled

The circumstance of being "homeless" provides numerous opportunities for "others" to determine the daily events of a mother's
life, options for change and the context of the mother/child relationship. "I don't feel like I control anything" was a pervasive expression among the mothers. The traditional role of mother as provider,
family leader, organizer and standard-setter was experienced by the
mothers as having vanished. Someone other than mother decided
when and where the family would rest, bathe or secure housing and
health care. Others determined what her family ate, evaluated her
abilities as a parent, judged her to need supportive services, parent
training or her fitness to retain custody of her children. If a mother
is determined by others to be using the daytime hours in unproduc-
tive or unmeaningful ways, she might be eliminated from the day

shelter program. If a mother or family received more than two meals a day in a shelter, they were determined to be ineligible for food stamps.

The mother's ability to re-establish order in her family and to reassert control over her life was often limited to the single and powerful use of the word *"no."* By saying a clear and confident *"no"* to bouncing basketballs, misbehaving children, or helpers, mothers took control from the "other." [The use of *"no"* as a verbal response, a silent or active behavior is not negative in the mother's experience.] The use of *"no"* by these mothers appears to be a creative and often positive resistance to dependence and external control. It reorders the hierarchy of daily living and relationships. It seems to be an active step toward regaining that which has been lost: an ordered mother/child relationship.

The extent to which each theme was manifest in the mothers' experience correlated with the mother's age. The younger the mother the more pronounced the frustration and dismay. In fact when the age of the oldest child is subtracted from the age of the mother, a case could be made for the effects of early pregnancy on limited acquisition of life skills, including parenting.

CONCLUSIONS

This article sets aside the psychiatric description of the population found by Bassuk (1986). The article presents instead a complementary description of relationships rather than an assessment of characteristics.

Data from this study clearly reveal that homelessness as a context for mother/child relationships forces an "out-of-order" relationship. It is important here to distinguish homelessness as a "circumstance" in which people use their energies to secure shelter from homelessness as a "context" for relationships. This study focuses on the latter. Homelessness as a context produces relationships which are lived-out in public. Mothers and children in this circumstance become public families, forced to engage in each and every task of daily living in full public view. The total spectrum of trivial to significant family action and interaction is open to public intervention. For these families, heretofore *private life*, i.e., eating, bathing, telephone conversation is now *public life with permission*.

Such a peculiar context for living leads the authors to refer to the mother/child relationship as "out-of-order" rather than "disordered." The absence of a home distorts the role of mother and child. Mothers lose opportunities to act as primary nurturers, teachers, negotiators and survival guides. A host of rotating volunteers, human service professionals and varied strange intruders (i.e., reporters, funding sources, researchers) assume with confidence and authority the functions normally and previously assumed by mothers.

As mothers become less assured of their abilities and opportunities to mother, children appear to become less confident and assured of their present and increasingly ambiguous about their future. The children experience uncomfortably divided loyalties. The adult/stranger provides the essentials of life: food, clothing, shelter, and often nurturance. The child is appreciative and hopeful for their permanence. The child is also aware that little is permanent except its mother. "With whom shall I play before bedtime?" becomes a critical question for the child. The only certain entity of tomorrow is mother. Yet the certainty of the moment is the volunteer. The natural mutuality of the mother/child relationship therefore is temporarily "out-of-order." The ways in which a mother can mother are limited. Likewise are the ways in which a child can "child." Psychologically or physically moving away from each other may mean getting one's needs met. Such movement, however, is always followed by moving toward each other for circumscribed safety. The stress and sadness of homelessness for these families creates an "out-of-order," a new context for their relationships.

IMPLICATIONS AND RECOMMENDATIONS

If the mother/child relationship can be considered "out-of-order" the implications for programming are strong.

1. Publicly supported day and night shelters would do well to reassess and strengthen the opportunities available for families to have private *time* if not *space*. We believe that any effort to

afford a family living in public a moment of privacy will enhance opportunities to restore order to their relationships. Whenever practical or possible, volunteers and professionals should encourage the creation of private moments in even the most public places.

2. The use of volunteers must be reassessed. Where volunteers are unintentionally replacing or usurping mothering roles this should be corrected and/or minimized. Consider meal, recreation and clean-up times as opportunities for the mother/child relationship to "re-order" itself naturally.

3. Children should be encouraged to feel less ambiguous about the elements of tomorrow. This can be accomplished through the "re-ordered" mother/child relationship and by the guided activity of volunteers. Every effort should be made to provide children with structured and unstructured, supervised and unsupervised opportunities to be affirmed and to express their feelings about their circumstance.

The authors do not suggest that every mother/child relationship among homeless women and children is "out-of-order." We know too well that "homelessness" is the homogeneous factor. However, we believe that based on these data the opportunities for "out-of-orderness" looms ever present among the total population.

Further study is needed to more clearly describe the experience of persons in this circumstance and the nature of relationships in such a context.

REFERENCES

Bassuk, E. (1986). Homeless Families: Single Mothers and Their Children in Boston Shelters. *The Mental Health Needs of Homeless Persons*. San Francisco: Jossey-Bass.

Bassuk, E., & Lauriat, A. (1986). Are Emergency Shelters The Solution? *International Journal of Mental Health*, 14(4), 72-97.

Bassuk, E. et al. (1986). Characteristics of Sheltered Homeless Families. *American Journal Public Health*, 76(9), 1097-1101.

Coliazzi, P. (1973). *Reflections and Research in Psychology*. Iowa: Kendall-Hunt Publishing Co.

Giorgi, A. (1970). *Psychology As A Human Science*. Harper and Row.

Patton, M. Q. (1975, February). *Alternative Evaluation Research Paradigm.* Grand Forks: University of North Dakota.

Rivlin, L. (1986). A New Look At The Homeless. *Social Policy*, 16(4), 3-10.

Rivlin, L. (1982). Group Membership And Place Meanings In A Urban Neighborhood. *Journal of Social Issues*, 38(3), 75-93.

Salerno, D. et al. (1984). *Hardship in The Heart Land: Homelessness in Eight American Cities.* New York: New York Community Service Society.

Wertz, F. S. Procedures In Phenomenological Research and The Question of Validity. *Studies in The Social Sciences.* (Carrollton, Georgia: West Georgia College). *23*, 29-47.

Homelessness Is Not Healthy
for Children and Other Living Things

James D. Wright

ABSTRACT. This chapter discusses the health problems of homeless children, youth, and women seen in the National Health Care
for the Homeless Program (HCH) during the program's first year.
On virtually all measures, homeless people—whether children or
adults, whether men or women—are more ill than their counterparts
in the domiciled ambulatory patient population; homelessness is indeed "unhealthy for children and other living things." Among children and youth, chronic physical disorders occur at approximately
twice the rate of occurrence among ambulatory children in general.
Pregnancies are noted as a special health problem; among HCH
women, more than a tenth have been pregnant at or since first contact with HCH, a pregnancy rate approximately twice that for US
women in general.

The last decade has apparently witnessed a substantial transformation of the homeless population of this nation. Whereas in previous decades the homeless were predominantly older, largely
white, broken-down alcohol-abusive men (or at least were stereoty-
pified as such), today a sizable fraction of the homeless consist of
women and children. This chapter discusses the effects of homelessness on the physical well-being of children, youth, and their
mothers.[1]

James D. Wright holds the Charles A. and Leo M. Favrot Chair in Human
Relations and is Professor in Sociology at Tulane University. He is the author of
numerous articles on health issues among the homeless population.

This research is supported by a grant from the Robert Wood Johnson Foundation (Princeton, NJ). Analyses, interpretations, and conclusions are the sole responsibility of the author.

65

The rationale for research on homelessness in general, or on various subgroups within the homeless population, is largely self-evident. In some fundamental respects, homelessness has become *the* social problem of the 1980s. (The only serious challenger would probably be AIDS.) Certainly, the large number of debilitated homeless persons wandering aimlessly over the landscapes of any of our major cities is shocking and offensive to the standards of decency that prevail in any civilized nation. That many of these people are now women and children, groups that society has traditionally obliged itself to protect, further offends our collective sensibilities. Skid Row drunks can be dismissed (correctly or otherwise) as largely beyond hope or in some sense personally responsible for their miseries. Homeless women fleeing an abusive family life, or who have lost their housing through abandonment by their male partners, or children living in station wagons because of the loss of parental employment, or who are themselves fleeing abusive family situations, cannot be so lightly dismissed. Indifference to the plight of homeless adult men comes easily in an illiberal era; indifference to the plight of homeless women, and especially homeless children, comes only to the mean-spirited.

The focus on the consequences of homelessness for physical health may seem less evident, but the rationale is again a strong one. Health problems are by no means the most serious problems homeless people face, ranking at least behind adequate shelter and nutrition on the agenda of human concerns. At the same time, attention to physical health may play an important role in attempts to address the many other problems homeless people face. Many homeless people are simply too ill to place in employment or other counselling programs, too ill to stand in line while their applications for benefits are being processed, too ill to search for housing within their means. The extreme poverty that characterizes the homeless population also severely limits their access to conventional health care, as does their general disaffiliation and estrangement from society and its institutions, health care institutions obviously included. Virtually all major cities have emergency shelters where anyone without housing can at least get out of the rain for the night; likewise, no city is without its soup kitchens and food banks where anyone who needs it can get a free meal. But where will a person with no home, no family, no medical insurance, and no money go to get health care?

Among the children in particular, poor physical health and especially chronic physical illness may well be found to contribute to the cycle of poverty, whereby the homeless children of today become the destitute and homeless adults of tomorrow. Chronically poor health or physical disabilities will at minimum interfere with, if not preclude, normal labor force participation, and with it, the ability to lead an independent adult existence. Thus, poor health may be one mechanism by which homelessness reproduces itself in subsequent generations.

In general, there is scarcely any aspect of a homeless existence that does not compromise physical health or at least greatly complicate the delivery of adequate health services; this, of course, is true of children no less than of adults. Life without adequate shelter is extremely corrosive of physical well-being. Minor health problems that most people would solve with a palliative from their home medicine cabinet become much more serious for people with no access to a medicine cabinet. Ailments that are routinely cured with a day or two at home in bed can become major health problems if one has neither home nor bed. One of the healthiest things Americans do every day is take a shower, a simple act of hygiene that is, perforce, largely denied to the homeless population.

The major features of a homeless existence that impact directly on physical well-being are an uncertain and often inadequate diet and sleeping location, limited or non-existent facilities for daily hygiene, exposure to the elements, direct and constant exposure to the social environment of the streets, communal sleeping and bathing facilities (for those fortunate enough to avail themselves of shelter), unwillingness or inability to follow medical regimens or to seek health care, extended periods spent on one's feet, an absence of family ties or other social support networks to draw upon in times of illness, extreme poverty (and the consequent absence of health insurance), high rates of mental illness and substance abuse, and a host of related factors (Brickner et al., 1985; Wright & Brickner, 1985). So far as the children specifically are concerned, there are additional complications. The shelters for women and children may well present optimal conditions for the transmission of infectious and communicable diseases to which children are especially prone (Gross & Rosenberg, 1987); a second problem is at least the possibility of widespread physical and sexual abuse. My purpose in this paper is to show how these "risk factors" impact upon the physical health of homeless children, youth, and women.

THE NATIONAL HEALTH CARE
FOR THE HOMELESS PROGRAM

In December 1984, the Robert Wood Johnson Foundation (Princeton, New Jersey) and the Pew Memorial Trust (Philadelphia, Pennsylvania), in conjunction with the United States Conference of Mayors, announced grants totalling $25 million to establish Health Care for the Homeless Programs in 19 major US cities.[2] Details on the background of this grant program and on program philosophy and configuration are reported elsewhere (Wright, 1987). Briefly, the program was conceived as "seed money," to get community-based health care for the homeless projects "up and running," with the strong expectation that each project would secure continuation funding from various federal, state, and local sources once the program grants expired. (The health care component of the recently enacted "Stuart B. McKinney Homeless Assistance Act" assures that most or all of the 19 HCH projects will in fact survive beyond the Johnson-Pew grant program.) Although there is wide variation among the 19 projects in approach, configuration, and specific program goals, all share a common and very strong community-based health care orientation. For the most part, the HCH projects are not sited in conventional health care settings; rather, they are located out in the community, in facilities utilized by the homeless population. Thus, HCH facilities are found in shelters, soup kitchens, missions, drop-in centers, alcohol detoxification facilities, juvenile court, and more or less anywhere else that homeless people are known to gather. Specific HCH health facilities run the entire gamut from fully equipped medical clinics on the one hand to little more than nursing stations on the other. All provide health care on demand to those of apparent need, without regard to health insurance or ability to pay. All projects also employ social workers and other human-services professionals to address needs that go beyond the strictly medical.

DATA

My research organization, the Social and Demographic Research Institute (SADRI), is funded by the Johnson Foundation to conduct research on the national HCH program. Again, details of the research design and data collection protocols are provided elsewhere (Wright, 1985; Wright et al. 1987). Briefly, each significant encounter between a homeless client and HCH staff generates a written medical note reported to us on a Contact Form. This form obtains limited demographic and other identifying information but is otherwise used as an open-ended progress note where care providers record their assessments of the client's problems and the treatment plan. Coding of the health information from these forms is done exclusively by registered nurses, using a modified version of the International Classification of Diseases (ICD) codes, ninth edition. All told, some 1200 codes are used to capture clients' physical health problems. These data form the basis for the following discussion.

Between program start-up and the end of March, 1987 (which represents about two years of program operation for the earliest-starting local projects and roughly five quarters of operation for the latest-starting projects), SADRI had received and processed about 173,000 Contact Forms representing contacts with some 59,000 distinct homeless individuals. As of this writing, our internal processing and checking of the Year II data are not yet completed; thus, the data reported here are derived from some 80,000 contacts with 30,000 people, which represents the documented program-wide client load through the end of June, 1986. For reasons discussed elsewhere (Wright et al., 1987), data from three of the nineteen project cities are also excluded here.

Although the majority (64%) of HCH clients have been adult men, a sizable minority (26%) have been adult women, and another sizable although smaller fraction (10%) have been homeless children (here defined as ages 15 and under).[3] If we add the late adolescents (ages 16 through 19) to the count, then the total proportion of women, children and youth increases to approximately three in eight. Thus, adult women and dependent children comprise more than a third of the client load. In some cities that work aggressively in shelters for women and children, these groups comprise well more than half the total.

The gender composition of HCH adults (among adults only, 29% are women and 71% are men) is very similar to that reported in other studies of the adult homeless population.[4] However, the heavy preponderance of men is true only of the adults; at all ages under 20, boys and girls appear in the data in approximately equal numbers. Compared to the adults, the children are somewhat likelier to be members of ethnic minorities (Blacks and Hispanics), but the difference is not large.

In general, homeless adult women are younger than homeless adult men; for example, 42% of the women but only 30% of the men are between the ages of 16 and 29. Otherwise, the two groups are very similar in their background characteristics (specifically, in ethnicity and educational attainment). The principal difference between them (other than age) is that about 25% of the adult women, but virtually none of the adult men, have dependent children in their care; a quarter of homeless women are in fact homeless mothers with children.

As to the children themselves (those under 16), they divide nearly equally between boys (49%) and girls (51%), as we have already said, and are heavily concentrated in the 1-4-year age category (54%). An additional third are in the 5-12-year old category, with the remainder (12%) being young adolescents (ages 13-15).

HEALTH PROBLEMS OF HOMELESS CHILDREN

Conventional notions of "childhood" and "adulthood" tend to break down in the context of homelessness in that many chronological children are forced to do very adult things. For our purposes, we have adopted an arbitrary cut-off at age 15 as demarcating the difference. It needs to be stressed, nonetheless, that not all of the children analyzed here are dependent children in the care of adults. Many of them, especially the young teenagers, are already "on their own," surviving independently of adult support. (The health

problems of homeless teenagers are addressed in a later section of
this paper.)

Selected health data for HCH children are shown in Table One,
both for the total and by gender. For reasons discussed elsewhere,
HCH data for persons seen only one time are generally not reliable;
all HCH data in this and subsequent tables are based only on clients
seen at least twice.[5] For comparison, the table also shows corres-

TABLE ONE

Occurrence of Selected Physical Disorders among HCH and NAMCS Children,
by Gender

	HCH			NAMCS		
	Total	Boys	Girls	Total	Boys	Girls
(N =)	1,028	532	496	6,055	3136	2,919
Per Cent Diagnosed With: [1]						
INFPAR	3.7	3.9	3.4	2.2	2.2	2.2
INF (Scabies, Lice)	7.3	6.4	8.3	0.2	0.3	0.2
NUTDEF	1.6	1.5	1.6	---	---	---
ANEMIA	2.2	1.3	3.2	1.1	1.1	1.1
NEURO	1.9	2.3	1.6	0.6	0.6	0.5
SEIZ	1.0	0.6	1.4	0.1	0.1	0.2
EYE	8.3	8.8	7.7	4.0	3.5	4.5
EAR	18.0	19.5	16.3	11.9	11.5	12.3
CARDIAC	2.8	2.8	2.8	0.5	0.5	0.5
MINURI	41.9	42.1	41.7	22.4	21.1	23.8
SERRI	2.8	4.1	1.4	2.2	2.1	2.2
GI	15.0	13.2	16.9	3.5	3.2	3.7
TEETH	4.5	5.6	3.2	0.4	0.5	0.3
PREG	---	---	3.6	---	---	---
SERSKIN	3.6	3.8	3.4	1.5	1.6	1.4
MINSKIN	19.8	18.8	21.0	5.4	4.8	6.0
PVD	1.9	2.3	1.6	0.6	0.7	0.6
ANYTRAUMA	10.2	9.6	10.3	7.0	8.5	5.4
ANYCHRO	15.4	16.5	14.1	8.8	9.2	8.2
ANYSTD	1.4	0.4	2.4	1.0	1.2	0.7

[1] See notes, Table Two, for definitions of the row labels. In this table,
children are clients with known dates of birth aged 15 or less. For the HCH
data, N = 16 cities, only children seen more than once.

ponding data for children included in the National Ambulatory Medical Care Survey (NAMCS). This survey was conducted in 1979 (the more recent 1985 version has not yet been released for analysis). Data for the survey were supplied by a national probability sample of ambulatory care physicians (N = 3,023); those in pediatric practice *were* included in the physician sampling frame. For each (or in large practices, for a systematic probability sample) of the ambulatory patients seen in a randomly stipulated week, the physicians filled out a short questionnaire giving limited background information and an account of principal health problems. Data for 46,351 ambulatory care patients were generated.[6]

NAMCS data shown in Table One are restricted to patients under age 16 living in the large urban areas (N = 6,055). These data are roughly comparable to the HCH data in two important senses: (1) both data sets describe *clinical* populations, that is, persons presenting at ambulatory clinics for attention to their health conditions, and (2) the medical information contained in both data sets has been provided by health care professionals. At the same time, the two data sets are grossly non-comparable in many other respects. The NAMCS data reported in this and subsequent tables may be taken as useful, heuristic reference points with which to compare the HCH experience, but these comparisons are not in any sense precise.

The general configuration of illness among homeless children is similar to that of children in general, although somewhat different than the configuration observed among homeless adults (acute disorders are more common, and chronic disorders less common, among the children than the adults). That is to say, the health problems faced by homeless children are not exotic or unusual disorders; they are, rather, the same health problems all children face. By far the most common disorders observed among the children are minor upper respiratory infections (approximately 40%), followed by minor skin ailments (approximately 20%), then ear disorders (mostly otitis media, at about 18%), then gastrointestinal problems (15%), and then trauma (about 10%), eye disorders (8%), and lice infestations (7%). In all these cases, differences in the rate of disorder between homeless boys and girls are minor.

Differences between homeless children and children in general, in contrast, are dramatic; although the general pattern of illness among homeless children is clearly not uncharacteristic of chil-dren's illnesses in general, the comparative rates of occurrence are inordinately high. Considering first the acute disorders: among NAMCS children, a mere 0.2% are found to have lice infestations, compared to more than 7% of the HCH children, a differential on the order of 35 to 1. Nutritional deficiencies are found among about 2% of the HCH children and are virtually non-existent among NAMCS children. Upper respiratory infections are twice as com-mon among homeless children as among ambulatory children in general, skin disorders about four times as common, GI disorders about four times as common, ear infections about twice as com-mon, poor dentition some ten times as common. Children, clearly, are not immune to the deleterious effects of homelessness on physi-cal well-being. That roughly half of these children are over age 5 and therefore required to attend school, where their illnesses can then circulate to other children, is an additional point of concern.

Differences in the rates of chronic physical disorders are even more disturbing. About 16% of the HCH children already have one or another chronic health condition: cardiac diseases (3%), anemia (2%), peripheral vascular disorders (2%), neurological disorders (2-3%), and so on.[7] The rate of chronic physical disorder among home-less children is nearly *twice* that observed among ambulatory chil-dren in general. The life chances of these children are obviously not bright to begin with; that they are already saddled with chronic dis-orders that may later prevent them from working and that will at least become life-long health problems further reduces their poten-tial for a productive and independent adult existence.

HEALTH PROBLEMS OF HOMELESS YOUTH

Table Two presents a somewhat more detailed view of the health problems of homeless youth, ages 13 through 19. The cell entries for this table are the same as in Table One; they show the percent-ages of HCH clients of various age-by-gender groupings who are afflicted with various health disorders. The columns represent nine different categories of homeless youth: 3 age groupings (13-15, 16-19, and, for comparison, those 20-24) by three gender groupings (young men, young women, and the age group total).

TABLE TWO

Health Problems of Homeless Youth

(N - 16 Cities, Clients Ages 13 to 24 Seen More than Once)

AGE GROUP	13 - 15			16 - 19			20 - 24		
GENDER	Boys	Girls	Total	Boys	Girls	Total	Boys	Girls	Total
N -	127	203	330	520	601	1121	1717	1051	2768

Percent Diagnosed With:

ACUTE PHYSICAL DISORDERS

INF	3.2	4.4	3.9	4.0	3.5	3.8	3.5	3.7	3.6
NUTDEF	0	1.0	0.6	1.2	2.5	1.9	0.9	1.0	0.9
OBESE	1.6	1.5	1.5	0.6	1.3	1.0	0.8	1.7	1.1
MINURI	22.8	26.1	24.9	34.8	22.1	28.0	24.6	23.5	24.2
SERURI	0.8	0	0.3	2.5	1.5	2.0	2.2	1.1	1.8
MINSKIN	13.4	9.4	10.9	12.9	8.0	10.3	11.5	9.2	10.6
SERSKIN	1.6	1.0	1.2	3.3	1.7	2.4	3.3	1.1	2.5
TRAUMA									
ANY	11.8	9.4	10.3	20.0	10.5	14.9	21.0	12.8	17.9
FX	0.8	0.5	0.6	2.5	1.0	1.7	3.4	1.4	2.6
SPR	3.9	3.0	3.3	7.3	3.3	5.2	7.1	3.7	5.8
BRU	3.2	2.5	2.7	3.7	4.0	3.8	4.1	4.7	4.3
LAC	4.7	4.4	4.6	9.4	2.8	5.9	6.9	3.5	5.6
ABR	1.6	1.0	1.2	1.9	0.5	1.2	2.5	0.8	1.8
BURN	0	0.5	0.3	1.0	0.7	0.8	1.1	0.4	0.8

CHRONIC PHYSICAL DISORDERS

ANYCHRO	15.0	11.8	13.0	16.2	12.0	13.9	16.7	14.3	15.8
CANC	0	0	0	0.4	0.2	0.3	0.2	0.1	0.2
ENDO	0	0.5	0.3	1.4	1.2	1.3	1.0	2.5	1.6
DIAB	0.8	0	0.3	0.6	0.2	0.4	0.7	0.6	0.7
ANEMIA	0.8	2.0	1.5	0.8	2.5	1.7	0.8	2.3	1.3
NEURO	3.2	1.0	1.8	4.8	4.2	4.5	3.9	6.1	4.7
SEIZ	0.8	0.5	0.6	1.7	1.3	1.5	1.6	1.3	1.5
EYE	8.7	6.9	7.6	5.8	5.0	5.4	4.5	3.5	4.1
EAR	5.5	1.5	3.0	4.4	4.0	4.2	3.5	4.4	3.8
CARDIAC	3.2	1.5	2.1	1.7	1.3	1.5	2.5	2.8	2.6
HTN	0.8	0.5	0.6	1.2	0.5	0.8	2.9	1.4	2.3
CVA	0	0	0	0	0	0	0	0	0
COPD	4.7	2.5	3.3	3.3	1.3	2.2	1.6	1.4	1.5
GI	6.3	9.4	8.2	6.5	9.3	8.0	8.7	10.6	9.4
TEETH	3.2	4.9	4.2	7.1	2.0	4.4	8.8	6.1	7.8
LIVER	0	0	0	1.0	0.7	0.8	0.6	0.4	0.5
GENURI	1.6	4.9	3.6	6.0	10.5	8.4	4.0	8.7	5.8
MALEGU	1.6	0	0.6	1.7	0	0.8	2.3	0	1.4
FEMGU	0	12.8	7.9	0	13.5	7.2	0	14.8	5.8
PREG	0	9.4	5.8	0	23.6	12.9	0	22.0	8.5
PVD	2.4	0.5	1.2	6.4	2.3	4.2	6.5	4.0	5.6
ARTHR	0	0	0	0.4	0.7	0.5	0.8	0.7	0.8
OTHMS	2.4	2.5	2.4	3.7	2.2	2.9	4.1	2.4	3.4

	13 - 15			16 - 19			20 - 24		
	Boys	Girls	Total	Boys	Girls	Total	Boys	Girls	Total
INFECTIOUS AND COMMUNICABLE DISORDERS									
AIDS/ARC	0	0	0	0	0	0	0.3	0	0.2
TB	0	0	0	0.2	0	0.1	0.2	0	0.1
PROTB	0	1.0	0.6	1.4	0.3	0.8	2.0	0.5	1.5
ANYTB	0	1.0	0.6	1.5	0.3	0.9	2.1	0.5	1.5
VDUNS	0	4.9	3.0	1.9	1.7	1.8	1.2	1.1	1.2
SYPH	0	0	0	0	0	0	0.2	0	0.1
GONN	0.8	3.4	2.4	1.7	1.2	1.4	1.1	1.5	1.3
ANYSTD	0.8	6.9	4.6	3.1	2.7	2.9	2.3	2.6	2.4
INFPAR	0	1.0	0.6	0.2	0	0.1	0.4	0.3	0.4
ANYPH	6.3	13.3	10.6	12.9	8.7	10.6	12.4	8.7	11.0

NOTES: Row labels are defined as follows:

Acute Disorders

INF	Infestational ailments (e.g., pediculosis, scabies, worms)
NUTDEF	Nutritional deficiencies (e.g., malnutrition, vitamin deficiencies)
OBESE	Obesity
MINURI	Minor upper respiratory infections (common colds and related symptoms)
SERRI	Serious respiratory infections not elsewhere classified (e.g., pneumonia, influenza, pleurisy)
MINSKIN	Minor skin ailments (e.g., sunburn, contact dermatitis, psoriasis, corns and callouses)
SERSKIN	Serious skin disorders (e. g., carbuncles, cellulitis, impetigo, abscesses)
TRAUMA	Injuries
ANY	Any trauma
FX	Fractures
SPR	Sprains and strains
BRU	Bruises, contusions
LAC	Lacerations, wounds
ABR	Superficial abrasions
BURN	Burns of all severities

Chronic Disorders

ANYCHRO	Any chronic physical disorder as defined in text.
CANC	Cancer, any site
ENDO	Endocrinological disorders (e.g., goiter, thyroid and pancreas disease)
DIAB	Diabetes mellitus
ANEMIA	Anemia and related disorders of the blood
NEURO	Neurological disorders, not including seizures (e.g., Parkinson's disease, multiple sclerosis, migraine headaches, neuritis, neuropathies)
SEIZ	Seizure disorders (including epilepsy)
EYE	Disorders of the eyes (e.g., cataracts, glaucoma, decreased vision)
EAR	Disorders of the ears (e.g., otitis, deafness, cerumen impaction)

TABLE TWO (continued)

CARDIAC	Heart and circulatory disorders, not including hypertension and cerebro-vascular accidents
HTN	Hypertension
CVA	Cerebro-vascular accidents/stroke
COPD	Chronic obstructive pulmonary disease
GI	Gastro-intestinal disorders (e.g., ulcers, gastritis, hernias)
TEETH	Dentition problems (predominantly caries)
LIVER	Liver diseases (e.g., cirrhosis, hepatitis, ascites, enlarged liver or spleen)
GENURI	General genito-urinary problems common to either sex (e.g., kidney, bladder problems, incontinence)
MALEGU	Genito-urinary problems found among men (e.g., penile disorders, testicular dysfunction, male infertility)
NOTE:	Data on MALEGU shown in the table are for males only in all cases.
FEMGU	Genito-urinary problems found among women (e.g., ovarian dysfunction, genital prolapse, menstrual disorders)
PREG	Pregnancies
NOTE:	Data on FEMGU and PREG shown in the table are for females only in all cases.
PVD	Peripheral vascular diseases
ARTHR	Arthritis and related problems
OTHMS	All musculo-skeletal disorders other than arthritis

Infectious and Communicable Disorders

AIDS/ARC	Autoimmune Deficiency Syndrome, AIDS-Related Complex
TB	Active tuberculosis infection, any site
PROTB	Prophylactic anti-TB therapeutic regimen
ANYTB	Either TB or PROTB or both
VDUNS	Unspecified venereal disease, herpes
SYPH	Syphilis
GONN	Gonorrhea
ANYSTD	Either VDUNS or SYPH or GONN, or any combination
INFPAR	Infectious and parasitic diseases (e.g., septicemia, diphtheria, tetanus, etc.)

Acute Disorders

As among the children, the predominant acute physical disorders suffered by HCH youth are upper respiratory infections, traumas, and minor skin disorders. Infestations (lice and scabies) are again quite common. In general, the boys are less healthy than the girls, although this pattern admits of several exceptions. Boys, particularly young men over age 16, show particularly high rates of injuries, especially sprains and lacerations. Except for trauma, there are no consistent effects for age shown in the table.

Chronic Physical Disorders

The proportion of HCH youth with any chronic physical disorder varies across the nine subgroups from 11.8% to 16.7% and averages 13.2%. This is again nearly twice the rate of chronic disease observed among those of equivalent age in the National Ambulatory Care Survey. In all age categories, chronic disorders are more common among males than females, although the difference is generally slight.

The most common chronic disorders observed among HCH youth are eye disorders (especially among the 13-15-year olds), gastrointestinal disorders (more common among girls than boys), ear problems, neurological impairments, problems with dentition (which increase with age over the range represented in the table), and genito-urinary problems (especially among those over 16 and among the young women). The rate of female GU problems is particularly high (8% for the 13-15-year olds, 14% for the 16-19-year olds, and 15% for those 20-24). Note also the astonishing rate of pregnancy among the girls: among those 13-15, 9.4% have been pregnant at or since their first contact with HCH; among those 16-19, the figure is 23.6% (the highest rate of pregnancy within *any* HCH age group); and among those 20-24, 22.0%. (Additional data on pregnancies are shown later.) Sexually transmitted diseases are accordingly also common (especially and somewhat surprisingly among the 13-15-year olds).[8]

Substance Abuse

Alcohol and drug abuse are for all practical purposes non-existent among the pre-teen homeless but do begin to be observed in children as young as 11 or 12. Indeed, among HCH clients aged 11-15, 6% of the boys and 7% of the girls are reported to have drug abuse problems; among those 16 to 19, drug abuse is observed among 16% of the young men and among 12% of the young women. The observed rate of drug abuse among 16-19-year-old HCH males is the highest to be found in any age grouping (Wright, 1987b: Table Two). As for alcohol abuse, the numbers are similar: among those 11-15, 11% of the boys and 8% of the girls have alcohol abuse problems; among those 16-19, the corresponding figures are 14% and 8% (Wright & Knight, 1987: 25).

We have *not* undertaken detailed disease-by-disease comparisons of these data with the NAMCS results for those ages 16-24; some preliminary analysis suggests that here as among the younger children, most disorders are at least twice as common among homeless youth as among ambulatory youth in general. With only a few exceptions, this is also true of homeless adults. This, of course, is scarcely a surprise: there is virtually no aspect of a homeless existence that does not impact deleteriously on a person's physical well-being, whatever their age or gender.

HEALTH PROBLEMS OF HOMELESS WOMEN

Table Three shows the rates at which various diseases and disorders have been observed among HCH adult clients, first for the total HCH client base, then for the subset of clients seen more than once, then separately for the adult men and women (seen more than once). As already stressed, about one woman in four is a homeless mother with a child or children in her care.

The first important point that surfaces in these data is that homeless adults in general are more ill than the domiciled ambulatory patient population on almost every indicator and usually by wide margins. That this is true has now been documented in a number of studies.[9] Indeed, the only apparent exceptions (in these data at least) are cancer, obesity, and stroke. The largest observed disparities (between the rates for homeless adults and those for the general ambulatory population) are in almost all cases directly referable to the conditions of the homeless existence: for example, upper respiratory infections, infestations (scabies and lice), skin disorders, virtually all categories of trauma, neurological disorders and seizures (resulting largely from the high rate of alcohol abuse among the homeless), gastrointestinal disorders, poor dentition, peripheral vascular disease, and tuberculosis. A summary indicator, the presence of any chronic physical disorder, shows that 41% of the HCH adults (seen more than once), but only 25% of the NAMCS patients, are afflicted with some chronic physical disability. Considering the apparently low rate of utilization of health services by the

TABLE THREE

Rates of Occurrence of Various Physical Disorders in the
HCH Adult Client Population

(N = 16 Cities, Adult Clients Only)

		HCH Clients			NAMCS Patients		
		Adults Seen More Than Once					
	All Adults	Total	Men	Women	Total	Men	Women
(N =)	23745	11886	8329	3468	28878		

ACUTE DISORDERS

Percent Diagnosed With:

INF	3.3	4.9	4.8	4.8	0.1	0.1	0.0
NUTDEF	1.2	1.9	1.7	2.4	0.1	0.1	0.1
OBESE	1.5	2.3	1.4	4.5	2.7	1.6	3.3
MINURI	23.6	33.2	33.4	32.8	6.7	7.0	6.6
SERRI	2.2	3.4	3.9	2.5	1.0	1.1	0.9
MINSKIN	9.8	13.9	14.1	13.5	5.0	5.4	4.7
SERSKIN	2.7	4.2	4.6	3.4	0.9	1.1	0.8
TRAUMA							
ANY	NA	23.4	26.3	16.7	NA	NA	NA
FX	3.1	4.5	5.4	2.5	2.2	3.2	1.6
SPR	5.1	7.1	7.6	5.9	3.1	4.2	2.5
BRU	4.0	5.6	5.7	5.3	1.0	1.4	0.7
LAC	6.3	8.6	10.5	4.3	1.2	2.1	0.6
ABR	1.5	2.2	2.6	1.3	0.4	0.5	0.3
BURN	0.8	1.1	1.2	0.8	0.2	0.3	0.1

CHRONIC DISORDERS

ANYCHRO	31.0	41.0	42.8	36.8	24.9	NA	NA
CANC	0.4	0.7	0.7	0.7	3.5	3.7	3.3
ENDO	1.4	2.2	1.5	3.8	1.6	0.9	2.0
DIAB	1.8	2.4	2.2	2.8	2.7	3.3	2.4
ANEMIA	1.3	2.2	1.7	3.5	0.9	0.7	1.0
NEURO	5.6	8.3	7.7	9.9	1.8	1.8	1.8
SEIZ	2.8	3.6	3.9	2.9	0.1	0.2	0.1
EYE	5.0	7.5	7.7	7.2	5.5	5.9	5.2
EAR	3.4	5.1	4.7	6.0	1.6	1.9	1.4
CARDIAC	4.4	6.6	6.9	5.7	6.2	7.9	5.2
HTN	10.4	14.2	15.7	10.8	8.0	8.0	8.1
CVA	0.1	0.3	0.3	0.1	0.7	0.9	0.5
COPD	3.2	4.7	4.8	4.4	3.2	4.2	2.7
GI	9.2	13.9	13.2	15.5	5.6	6.2	5.2
TEETH	7.0	9.3	9.7	8.6	0.3	0.3	0.3
LIVER	0.9	1.3	1.5	1.0	0.3	0.4	0.2
GENURI	4.1	6.6	4.2	12.4	2.9	2.3	3.2
MALEGU	1.3	1.9	1.9	----	3.2	3.2	---
FEMGU	11.3	15.8	---	15.8	7.3	---	7.3

TABLE THREE (continued)

	All Adults	Total	Men	Women		Total	Men	Women
PREG	9.9	11.4	---	11.4		0.5	---	0.5
PVD	9.1	13.1	14.0	11.1		0.9	1.3	0.7
ARTHR	2.7	4.2	4.1	4.3		3.7	3.4	3.8
OTHMS	3.9	6.0	6.3	5.3		5.8	6.6	5.3
			INFECTIOUS AND COMMUNICABLE DISORDERS					
AIDS/ ARC	0.1	0.2	0.2	0.1		NA	NA	NA
TB	0.3	0.5	0.6	0.2		0.1	0.1	0.1
PROTB	2.5	4.5	5.4	2.5		NA	NA	NA
ANYTB	2.7	4.9	5.8	2.7		NA	NA	NA
VDUNS	0.4	0.7	0.7	0.7		0.6	0.8	0.5
SYPH	0.1	0.2	0.2	0.2		0.1	0.1	0.0
GONN	0.5	0.8	0.6	1.3		0.1	0.1	0.0
ANYSTD	NA	1.6	1.4	2.0		NA	NA	NA
INFPAR	0.2	0.3	0.4	0.3		0.7	0.8	0.6

Notes:

(1) Columns

The first column of numbers shows data for all HCH adult clients ever seen (N - 16 cities), regardless of number of contacts.

The next three columns of numbers show data for adult clients seen more than once (N - 16 cities), first for the total, then by gender.

The last three columns of numbers shows corresponding data for adult respondents in urban areas from the National Ambulatory Medical Care Survey, first for the total, then by gender.

(2) Rows

The top row in each table gives sample sizes for each relevant group. Acronyms used to define the remaining row entries are defined as in Table Two.

(3) Cell Entries

Cell entries show the percentage of various groups who have been diagnosed with the various disorders shown in the rows. NA - not available at this time.

homeless in the absence of targeted programs such as HCH, these data therefore suggest that the homeless may well harbor the largest pool of untreated disease left in this country.[10]

The unique health problems of homeless adult women can be seen in either of two comparisons: in the comparison with homeless adult men and in the comparison with NAMCS women. Concerning the second of these, the picture is largely the same as that for children and youth: in most cases, the rates of all disorders examined in the table are higher, and often much higher, than corresponding rates among NAMCS women. Like homeless persons in general, homeless women are more physically ill than their counterparts in the general population.

The comparison between homeless adult women and homeless adult men is rather more interesting. In the general literature on gender differences in health status, the principal generalization is "more morbidity among women, more mortality among men." (This literature is reviewed in Lam, 1987). Rephrased slightly, the pattern is that women tend to report (or to exhibit) elevated rates of the less serious disorders, while men show elevated rates of the more serious disorders, the so-called "killer diseases" (and, of course, have shorter life expectancies). Among the homeless, these differences are greatly attenuated. Indeed, in most cases, the rates for homeless women and men are practically identical. The principal exceptions are that (1) homeless men are clearly at higher risk for tuberculosis, hypertension, and for all categories of trauma than are homeless women (as in the general population), (2) homeless women show higher rates of eating and related nutritional disorders (nutritional deficiencies, obesity, anemia), (3) homeless women show higher rates of endocrinological disorders and, to a lesser extent, diabetes, and (4) homeless women have strongly elevated rates of genito-urinary disorders. Many of the gender differences routinely reported in studies of domiciled men and women apparently disappear among the homeless.[11]

We have already noted that, on average, HCH women are younger than HCH men, a fact with some possible health consequences. As it happens, the women are also *much* less alcohol-abusive (roughly by a factor of three) but exhibit *higher* rates of mental illness (roughly by a factor of two) (Wright et al., 1987; Wright & Knight, 1987).[12] A series of multivariate analyses (data not shown) reveals that when these factors are held constant, the gender differences among HCH clients are further reduced. Net of these other factors, men continue to show elevated rates of trauma and hypertension, and women continue to show elevated rates of GI disorders and genito-urinary problems; the male-female differences in the other cases examined are not statistically significant.[13]

The preceding run of results summarizes easily: homeless people, whether men or women, whether children or adults, are physically more ill than their counterparts in the general population; homeless men and women are, with a few exceptions, about equally ill, presumably because the condition of homelessness itself simply overwhelms most other factors.

PREGNANCIES

One unique health problem faced by homeless women is pregnancy, whether wanted or unwanted. The average age of homeless people (in this and many other studies) is reliably reported to be in the early to middle thirties. It is therefore to be expected that they are a sexually active group, a point that nonetheless surprises many people, perhaps because the stereotypical image of the homeless is that they are too broken-down to sustain any degree of sexuality. And yet, as indicated in Table Three, 11.4% of the adult HCH women (seen more than once) have been pregnant at or since their first contact with HCH, a surprisingly high percentage.

How does this rate of pregnancy compare to that of US women in general? Unfortunately, national statistical series do not keep track of pregnancies, only of live births. The annual national birthrate is approximately 15 live births per 1000 population, or 30 per 1000 women (= 3%) (Westoff, 1986); thus, the annual rate of pregnancy among adult US women could not possibly exceed five or six per cent. It would therefore appear that the rate of pregnancies among adult HCH women is some two times the national rate.

What accounts for this difference? One possibility is a higher rate of sexual promiscuity among homeless women, but the data fail to bear this out. If it were a matter of more promiscuous sexuality, we would expect to find equally elevated rates of sexually transmitted infections. The data in Table Three show 187 cases of sexually transmitted infection (syphilis, gonorrhea, and other unspecified STDs) among 11,886 HCH adults (seen more than once), which translates to a rate of 1,573 infections per hundred thousand homeless adults. The latest data from the Centers for Disease Control (CDC, 1985) show a rate of sexual infection in the adult population at large of 1,403 per hundred thousand, a negligible difference compared to the apparent difference in the pregnancy rate. A more plausible explanation of the pregnancy differential would therefore apparently involve limited knowledge about or access to contraception, or possibly, a high incidence of pregnancy resulting from rape.[14] Unfortunately, we have no direct way of testing these possibilities in our data.

Table Four shows the percentage of HCH adult women of various age groups who have been pregnant at or since their first contact with HCH, separately for whites and non-whites. The highest rate of pregnancy is found among the youngest (16-19-year old) cohort, among whom about a quarter have been pregnant during their contact with HCH; the rate exceeds 20% for the next oldest cohort (ages 20-24), exceeds 10% for the following cohort (ages 25-29), and then drops off quickly. White-nonwhite differences are trivial in all age categories.

As it happens, pregnant women tend to exit the HCH system rather rapidly, being referred off in most cases to more appropriate

TABLE FOUR

Pregnancies among Adult HCH Women by Age and Race

(N - 16 Cities, Only for Adult Women Seen More than Once)

	Percentage Pregnant					
Age Group	All HCH Women		White Women		Nonwhite Women	
	%	N	%	N	%	N
16 - 19	23.6	601	24.1	294	23.4	286
20 - 24	22.0	1051	21.6	473	21.7	538
25 - 29	11.9	1193	12.0	500	11.5	668
30 - 34	8.1	1017	8.2	389	7.6	595
35 - 45	3.7	1448	3.6	658	3.9	735
46 +	0.1	1407	0.1	833	--	531

Note: Cell entries show the percentages of women clients (of varying age and ethnic characteristics) who were pregnant at first contact or who have become pregnant since first contact, not the percentages ever pregnant.

prenatal care programs (Wright et al., 1987: 21-22). We therefore have little information on pregnancy outcomes, and no information at all on the newborn's situation at birth (e.g., birth weight, congenital disorders, etc.) We do know that among the 395 pregnancies registered among HCH adult women seen more than once, at least 31 were not carried to term (16 known miscarriages, 15 induced abortions). The fate of the remaining 364 pregnancies is, unfortunately, unknown.

CONCLUSIONS

Homeless persons of all genders and ages are exposed to, and therefore exhibit, a characteristic "package" of disorders that are directly and immediately referable to the conditions of a homeless existence. Among the acute disorders, this package includes upper respiratory infections, skin ailments, lice infestations, and trauma of all sorts; among the more chronic disorders, the package includes peripheral vascular disease, tuberculosis, GI disorders, poor dentition, and others. Among homeless women, problems related to pregnancy must be added to the list; among the children, one would add ear infections as well. The health problems of the homeless population are further complicated by the lack of access to medical care, poor compliance with treatment regimen, and generally unsanitary and unsafe living conditions, along with a host of other factors.

Part of the differentially poor health observed among homeless adults is due to the atypical demographic configuration of the group—it is a result of the homeless being largely male, disproportionally non-white, and extremely poor. Yet another part is ascribable to the high rates of substance abuse, particularly alcohol abuse. These points notwithstanding, multivariate analyses controlling for these (and other) factors show rather decisively that the key factor in the ill health of the homeless—whether children or adults—is not demographics and not substance abuse: the key factor is homelessness itself (Knight, 1987). Among the many good reasons to "do something" about homelessness is that homelessness makes people ill—it is unhealthy for children, for their parents, and for other living things. In the extreme, it is a fatal condition.[15]

NOTES

1. In point of fact, women and children have always comprised a sizable portion of the American homeless population, from Colonial times to the present. Historical data on homeless women are reviewed in some detail in Lam (1987: Ch. Two).

2. The 19 participating cities are: Albuquerque, Baltimore, Birmingham, Boston, Chicago, Cleveland, Denver, Detroit, Los Angeles, Milwaukee, Nashville, Newark, New York City, Philadelphia, Phoenix, San Antonio, San Francisco, Seattle, and Washington, DC.

3. The sample size for the above calculations is 25,068. This excludes clients whose age is not known and a smaller number whose gender is not known.

4. See Knight and Lam, 1987. Over a range of recent (post-1980) studies, the average proportion of women among homeless adults is around 20-25%, very close to the HCH figures.

5. See Wright et al., 1987: 22-29. The problem in essence is that many of the one time contracts are very fleeting encounters that do not provide an opportunity to probe in detail into a client's health problems. In point of fact, the rates of virtually every disorder we have examined tend to increase as the number of client contacts increases, up to about four or five contacts, at which point the rates level off. Part of this effect is presumably substantive: sicker people return to clinic more often. Our analysis suggests, however, that the larger share of the effect is methodological: clients need to be seen a relatively large number of times before a complete and reliable health picture can be obtained.

6. A full account of methods and technical details for the NAMCS survey is given in Public Health Service, *National Ambulatory Medical Care Survey: Background and Methodology*. Vital and Health Statistics Series 2, Number 61 (1979).

7. A client is considered to have a chronic physical disorder in this analysis if any of the following health problems are present (either by diagnosis or history): tuberculosis; prophylactic TB therapy; AIDS; cancer (any site); diabetes mellitus; anemia; seizure disorders; seriously impaired vision or hearing; cardiovascular disease, including stroke, hypertension; chronic obstructive pulmonary disease; liver disease; arterial disease; all colostomies; kidney disease; chronic peripheral vascular disease; all tracheotomies; amputations (other than fingers and toes); and paraplegia. The same definition applies to NAMCS patients as well.

8. Unfortunately, our data do not allow us to differentiate between youth who are homeless and on the streets with their families vs. those who are already out "on their own." Our *impression* is that most of the 16-and-over homeless youth are already independent of their families, whereas at least some of the 13-15-year olds are not. Not all of the youth shown here, in short, are "runaway" or "throwaway" kids, although, without doubt, many are.

9. See, e.g., Bassuk (1984); Bassuk et al., 1986); Brickner et al., (1985); Jonas (1986); Rossi et al., (1987); US Conference of Mayors (1985); Wright et al., 1987; 1987b); etc.

10. A recent study of homeless persons seeking care in St. Louis reports that

more than 70% had *no* usual health care provider and that more than half had not received any health care attention in the previous year (Healthcare for the Homeless Coalition of Greater St. Louis, 1986). It is widely reported that the principal sources of health care for the homeless are hospital emergency rooms, which further implies that homeless people rarely seek care until their condition has degenerated to emergency status. See, for example, Elvy (1985), and the references therein. That the poor in general encounter formidable obstacles in accessing appropriate health care is very well-documented (see, e.g., Freeman, 1987; L. Aday, G. V. Fleming, and R. Anderson, 1984; that the problems encountered by the homeless are any less profound is inconceivable.

11. Why might this be the case? Although a number of hypotheses might be entertained, the most plausible (in our view) is that the condition of homelessness simply overpowers most gender factors in determining health differences. Many of the "killer diseases" that are found to be more common among men than among women are often attributed to differential levels of stress, at least as a contributory factor. It is certainly conceivable that the condition of homelessness is equally stressful for men and women, thereby reducing or eliminating the difference. That women, by tradition, are "in the home" whereas men are "in the workplace" is also regularly cited as a factor in gender differences in health among the general population; the day-to-day lives of homeless men and homeless women, of course, exhibit no such patterns.

12. Our estimates are that about 48% of the adult men, and about 16% of the adult women, are alcohol-abusive; likewise, about 40% of the women and about 20% of the men show some psychiatric impairment other than alcohol abuse.

13. It is of particular significance that the zero-order difference in "any chronic disease" (37% of the HCH women and 43% of the HCH men) disappears entirely with other factors controlled. A detailed look at the regression results makes it quite plain that the initial difference is due exclusively to the higher rate of alcohol abuse among HCH men. See Wright and Knight (1987) for a more extended discussion of these data.

14. Kelly (1985:87) has reported that the rate of sexual assault on homeless women is approximately 20 times the rate among women in general, and so this hypothesis is not to be lightly dismissed.

15. We know of only two studies of mortality among the homeless. One is based on Swedish data (Alstrom, Lindelius & Salum, 1975) and showed an excess mortality among the homeless amounting to a factor of four; over the period studied, that is, the number of observed deaths exceeded the number of expected deaths by four times. The average age at death was about 53 years. Our own analysis of deaths occurring among HCH clients showed a similar mortality excess, with the average age at death being about 51 years. Twenty-six per cent of the deaths occurring to HCH clients, incidentally, are the result of homicide; in the general US population, homicide accounts for about 1% of the annual deaths. See Wright and Weber (forthcoming) for details.

REFERENCES

Aday, L., Fleming, G. V., & Anderson, R. (1984). *Access to Medical Care in the US: Who Has It, Who Doesn't* (Chicago, Pluribus Press).

Alstrom, C. H., Lindelius, R., & Salum, I. (1975). "Mortality among Homeless Men." *British Journal of Addiction* 70: 245-252.

Bassuk, E. (1984). "The Homeless Problem." *Scientific American* 251(1): 40-45.

Bassuk, E., Rubin, L., & Lauriat, A. (1986). "Characteristics of Sheltered Homeless Families." *American Journal of Public Health* 76(9): 1097-1101.

Brickner, P. W., Scharer, L.K., Conanan, B., Elvy, A., & Savarese, M. (Eds.). (1985). *Health Care of Homeless People* (New York: Springer).

Centers for Disease Control (CDC). (May, 1985) "Summary—Cases of Specific Notifiable Diseases, United States, Table One." *Morbidity and Mortality Weekly Report* (31 May).

Elvy, A. (1985). "Access to Care," Ch. 16 (pp. 223-231) in P. W. Brickner et al., *Health Care of Homeless People* (New York: Springer).

Freeman, H. et al. (1987). "Americans Report on Their Access to Care." *Health Affairs* 6:1 (Spring), pp. 6-18.

Gross, T. P. & Rosenberg, M. L. (1987). "Shelters for Battered Women and Their Children: An Underrecognized Source of Communicable Disease Transmission." *American Journal of Public Health* 77:9 (September), pp. 1198-1201.

Healthcare for the Homeless Coalition of Greater St. Louis (1986). *Program Description*, Report.

Jonas, S. (1986). "On Homelessness and the American Way." *American Journal of Public Health* 76(9): 1084-1086.

Kelly, J. T. (1985). *Alcohol Abuse Among the Homeless*. Unpublished doctoral dissertation, Department of Sociology, University of Massachusetts, Amherst.

Knight, J. W. & Lam, J. (1987). "Health and Homelessness: A Review of the Literature." Unpublished ms., Social and Demographic Research Institute, University of Massachusetts.

Lam, J. (1987). *Homeless Women in America: Their Social and Health Characteristics*. Unpublished doctoral dissertation, Department of Sociology, University of Massachusetts, Amherst.

Rossi, P. H., Wright, J.D., Fisher, G., & Willis, G. (1987). "The Urban Homeless: Estimating Composition and Size." *Science* 235 (4794) (13 March): 1336-1341.

US Conference of Mayors (1985). *Health Care for the Homeless: A Forty City Review* (Washington, DC: US Conference of Mayors).

Westoff, C. (1986). "Fertility in the United States." *Science* 234 (31 October), pp. 554-559.

Wright, J. D. (1985). "The 'Health Care for the Homeless' Program: Evaluation

88   *Homeless Children: The Watchers and the Waiters*

Design and Preliminary Results." Paper read at the Annual Meeting of the American Public Health Association (Washington, DC) (November).

Wright, J.D. (1987). "The National Health Care for the Homeless Program." Ch. 9 in Bingham, Green and White (eds)., *The Homeless in Contemporary Society* (Newbury Park, CA: Sage Publications).

Wright, J.D. (1987b). *Selected Topics in the Health Status of America's Homeless.* A Special Report to the Institute of Medicine, National Academy of Sciences (Amherst, MA: SADRI0.)

Wright, J. D. & Brickner, P. W. (1985). "The Health Status of the Homeless: Diverse People, Diverse Problems, Diverse Needs." Paper read at the Annual Meetings of the American Public Health Association (Washington, DC) (November).

Wright, J. D. & Knight, J. W. (1987). *Alcohol Abuse in the National Health Care for the Homeless Client Population.* Washington, DC: National Institute on Alcohol Abuse and Alcoholism.

Wright, J. D. & Weber, E. (forthcoming). *Homelessness and Health.* New York: McGraw Hill Publishing Company.

Wright, J. D., Weber-Burdin, E., Knight, J., & Lam, J. (1987). *The National Health Care for the Homeless Program: The First Year.* Amherst, MA: Social and Demographic Research Institute.

Wright, J. D., Rossi, P. H., Knight, J. W., Weber-Burdin, E., Tessler, R., Steward, C., Geronimo, J., & Lam, J. (1987b). "Homelessness and Health: Effects of Life Style on Physical Well Being Among Homeless People in New York City." Pp. 41-72 in M. Lewis and J. Miller (eds), *Research on Social Problems and Public Policy*, Volume IV, 41-72. Greenwood CT: JAI Press.

Homeless Children:
A New Vulnerability

Mark Rosenman, PhD
Mary Lee Stein, MSW

ABSTRACT. Using Washington, D.C. as an exemplar of urban programs for homeless children, the authors define current service gaps and public policy failures. The article calls attention to the varied social service needs of the population and points the reader toward action steps which may channel good intentions and public interest into real and measurable change.

INTRODUCTION

Growing numbers of our children, including many who previously enjoyed a seemingly secure middle-class life, are faced with a dramatic new kind of vulnerability. They are homeless. They are not falling through holes in the "safety net" — they miss it. It is not set up in such a way as even to check their fall. A major study found that "Families comprise the largest group for whom emergency shelter and other needed services are particularly lacking . . ." (Reyes & Waxman, 1986, p. 15).

According to available data, there are over 500,000 children nationally (other estimates go as high as 800,000) who remain in the

Mark Rosenman is Director of the Institute for Public Policy of the Union for Experimenting Colleges and Universities (UECU). He is also a professor in the UECU's nonresidential PhD program, the Union Graduate School. Dr. Rosenman has a long history of work at the interface of education and social change. Mary Lee Stein is a clinical social worker in a therapeutic nursery operated in a public elementary school by the District of Columbia's Commission on Mental Health. She is an associate of the UECU Institute for Public Policy. Ms. Stein has considerable experience in working with inner-city families and their children.

care of at least one biological parent, but who have no home (Dobbins, 1987; Martin, 1987). It also has been suggested that 25% of the single adult homeless have children whom they placed temporarily with relatives or friends before seeking public shelter alone (Lane & Depp, 1987). Without even counting those children, more than 35% of the homeless nationally are in families (Melnick & Williams, 1987) and they constitute the fastest growing portion of the homeless population (Reyes & Waxman, 1986). Their numbers are increasing on an average of 20% to 30% a year (Waxman & Reyes, 1987; Reyes & Waxman, 1986).

The problem is expected to grow much worse fairly quickly. One estimate found that in 1983 there were 11.9 million low-income families unable to find affordable housing and in danger of becoming homeless (Whitman & Bosc, 1987). Another study estimates that there will be 18 million homeless people in the U.S. within about 15 years (Clay, cited in Jordan, 1987). Today in the U.S. there are over 2 million people without assurance of sleeping quarters for the next thirty days (Rivlin, 1986).

One study estimates that today fully 20% of all poor children in the United States are experiencing homelessness at some time in their lives (Melnick & Williams, 1987). Just short of public homelessness are the thousands and thousands of additional families forced to double-up and triple-up with relatives and friends (Waxman & Reyes, 1987; Whitman & Bosc, 1987). Over 50% of all homeless families had lived with friends and relatives before being forced to seek public shelter; 75% of them have been homeless for more than three months (Maza & Hall, 1986). They have brought a new term—*couch people*—into common usage (Whitman & Bosc, 1987).

Simply put, the problem of homeless families is becoming astronomical. The plight of these hundreds of thousands of homeless children must be called a national shame.

Beyond the occasional news story of a homeless family living in a parked car, we hear little of these children. The popular image of homelessness is an adult "street person" sleeping on heating grates in winter, off in a corner of some park in warmer weather. We tend not to think of the thousands upon thousands of at least partially intact families moving from street to shelter and back again, searching for some form of sanctuary. Yet, increasingly they are the homeless.

While many homeless families are grounded in a history of poverty, their numbers are being swelled by those of middle-class background. More and more of the homeless are among those unable to escape growing threats to the security of middle-class life. Newspaper stories begin to chronicle events such as a family of four with a $35,000 wage earner reduced to an $18,000 income because of a job-related back injury, foundering under obligations which assumed a continued salary, and suddenly rendered homeless (Collier, 1986). It is very interesting to note, for example, that *almost 20% of homeless adults are employed* (Reyes & Waxman, 1986).

The situation and problems, the new vulnerability, of these families and children are not well addressed by existing government programs. Homelessness is not simply one more issue which must be faced by children and the agencies serving them. It is an overriding and extraordinarily disruptive circumstance. It goes well beyond creating another category of "need." It significantly complicates life and adversely impacts on every attempt to respond to any and all needs of such children.

PROBLEMS OF HOMELESS CHILDREN AND FAMILIES

The problems confronted by homeless families and children are myriad and profound. As one study put it, they represent a horrendous "interconnectedness between societal neglect and personal misfortune" (Melnick & Williams, 1987, p. 4).

The obvious root cause of homelessness is the absence of affordable housing, a point noted over and over again in most studies of the problem (e.g., Flynn, 1987; Reyes & Waxman, 1986; Melnick & Williams, 1987) and one to which we will return later. Other immediate factors often cited as causes of homelessness include unemployment, underemployment and low-wage employment, substance abuse and lack of treatment opportunities, mental illness and lack of treatment opportunities, domestic violence and lack of refuge and services, inadequate income maintenance programs, population shifts, and (related to housing) involuntary evictions (Reyes & Waxman, 1986). It is interesting to note, for example, that fully two-thirds of homelessness in the District of Columbia is caused by evictions (Melnick & Williams, 1987).

Before looking at the specific needs of these families and children, it is important first to understand some of the dynamics which they face beyond the factors causing their homelessness. "Homelessness leads to a breakdown of family unity and stability which results in fragmentation and dependency." "The impact of homelessness on families is cumulative and very destructive" (Waxman & Reyes, 1986, p. 10). In other words, homelessness not only compounds its originating difficulties, but itself frustrates remedy and the family's ability to cope with its own problems.

Homelessness creates a context which is problematic beyond the quest for shelter and sanctuary. Without understanding those contextual issues, the most well intentioned of social welfare efforts will miss its mark.

To provide insight into the full dimensions of children's homelessness we will look first at what is needed, and then later at what must be done to augment the parent's (parents') ability to meet the needs of children. We build on accepted understandings of children's needs, a sense of services now being provided in relation to them, and look at the ways the multitude of problems created by poverty (even for those only temporarily facing hard times) are compounded by homelessness.

Shelter and Family Cohesion

Beyond the other strains of homelessness on family cohesion noted below, parents with children often experience difficulty in finding shelter together. Such facilities are in shortest supply in serving various categories of the homeless (Reyes & Waxman, 1986). One estimate is that more than 30% of those families *requesting* shelter are turned away (Waxman & Reyes, 1987). Another estimate suggests that fewer than one in three needing shelter comes in from the streets (Robinson, 1985).

It is reported that many homeless families needing shelter never request it out of fear that their children will be taken away from them (Waxman & Reyes, 1987). In some locales parents are threatened, by the very agencies that are supposed to be helping them, with the "removal" of their children because of their failure to provide suitable housing (Reyes & Waxman, 1986).

The inadequacy of current resources would be exponentially greater if all families needing shelter were to demand it. Even in some communities required by local law and federal regulation to provide such service, the response is inadequate to the need (*Russell, Seabook, Father McKenna Center and National Coalition for the Homeless v. Barry, Hawkins & Bowen*, 1987).

The fear of family dissolution is not groundless. Family members sometimes are forced to separate from one another in order to obtain shelter. One study of urban areas reported that in two-thirds of the cities, families are in fact broken up as the price of shelter (Waxman & Reyes, 1987). Other times families have been forced to produce documentation of marriage and parenthood/guardianship as prerequisite to being sheltered together (*Russell et al. v. Barry et al.*, 1987).

Once parents and children find a place in a shelter, their problems are not over. Beyond the constellation of difficulties addressed below is the fact that most cities limit shelter stays for any particular family. The general rule appears to be about a month for emergency shelter and an additional two months for "transitional shelter" (Waxman & Reyes, 1987). This is problematic since more than 75% of these families are homeless for considerably longer than three months (Maza & Hall, 1986).

It is reported that many cities charge a fee for sheltering parents and children, in part because they fear that no matter how inadequate the facilities, families might tend to become too dependent (D. Pavetti, personal communication, September 28, 1987). The Reagan administration recently established regulations requiring that the value of shelter, food, etc., provided by charity to homeless families and children receiving Supplemental Security Income be deducted from that support; these regulations were withdrawn under congressional pressure (Associated Press, 1987).

Schooling

Numerous studies have found major difficulties being confronted by homeless children of school age. One found that children are denied access to their regular school when they are sheltered outside of its district boundaries, and often are denied access to schools serving the shelter's district because of the temporary nature of their residence in it. They are denied school transportation, needed special classes, and other services (Center for Law and Education, 1987). Even homeless children residing temporarily with relatives and family friends are denied school enrollment unless parental guardianship has been surrendered (Homeless Persons Survival Act, 1986). News stories chronicle homeless children *denied any schooling* by such "Catch 22's" (Winerip, 1987).

As a result of such problems, another study found that 43% of school-age homeless children are not attending school at all (Center for Law and Education, 1987). Still another report found additional major problems of irregular attendance, failing and below-grade performance (43% had been forced to miss one grade), and an unusual need for special education classes (Bassuk, Rubin & Lauriat, 1986). Dropping-out, truancy, unstable attendance and lowered achievement are associated with the stigmatization of being a homeless child ridiculed by peers (Waxman & Reyes, 1987).

The chief social worker/manager of a large public shelter (Capital City Inn, Washington, D.C.) observes that the simple absence of laundry facilities or the money to have clothes cleaned means that some parents feel forced to keep their children home from school (E. McCall, personal communication, September 18, 1987). Others are unable to finance school transportation for their children. Silvan Alleyne (now teaching at Howard University) noted from interviews of homeless families that many parents are reluctant to register children using a shelter as their address (personal communication, October 8, 1987).

Psychosocial Development and Mental Health

Homeless children exhibit an extraordinary range and scale of emotional problems. They are found to be higher than their peers in shyness, dependent behavior, aggression, attention deficiencies, withdrawal and demanding behavior (Bassuk et al., 1986). They demonstrate increased stress, anxiety and depression, as well as significantly lowered self-esteem (Waxman & Reyes, 1987). It is reported that a majority of homeless children over the age of five acknowledge suicidal feelings (Haddock, 1986).

Some experts on homelessness, such as Tony Russo (1987), executive director of the Consortium for Services to Homeless Families (CONSERVE, located in Washington, D.C.), note that homeless children will present with a "flat affect" (personal communication, May 11, 1987). Russo reports maladaptive behavior, alarmingly slowed cognitive development, hyperactivity and a great deal of angry, aggressive behavior. His suspicion that these children also experience developmental delays, developmental regression, and other stress-related symptoms and illnesses is affirmed by studies (Waxman & Reyes, 1987; Bassuk et al., 1986).

Physical Health

Homeless children, more than their peers, suffer from poor health and a variety of physical illness; personal hygiene deteriorates under shelter conditions (Waxman & Reyes, 1987). One observer notes a tendency for minor, but often significant, illnesses and ailments to go untreated, with mostly only emergency health needs being addressed (Alleyne, personal communication, 1987).

Nutrition

Adequate diet is a problem for homeless children (Bassuk et al., 1986; Rowe, 1986). Many shelters have no cooking facilities or feeding programs (Kurtz, 1987). The cost of food, whether the homeless are forced to buy prepared meals or to purchase food and try to cook themselves, is limited by federal subsidy to under $1 (seventy-one cents) per person per meal (Kurtz, 1987). Even the preparation and heating of a baby's formula can pose extraordinary hardships. Most shelters do not provide families with the facilities to store food, or even to keep milk and formula refrigerated (Russo, 1987).

Infants

Few shelters will even accept infants (Homeless Persons' Survival Act, 1986). Those that do fail to help parents provide the stimulation so necessary to their development. Russo (1987) suspects profoundly stunted growth and lack of responsiveness in infants under two years of age and sees limited physical, cognitive, speech and language development. McCall (1987) says that the greatest unmet need of sheltered families with very young children is for good infant care, infant stimulation programs, and help in developing parenting skills in young (sometimes teenage) parents.

Peer Relationships

Children are the "silent victims" of homelessness: "They are not able to make friends with anyone; they are always 'strangers.'" (Waxman & Reyes, 1987). The friendships so essential to normal childhood development elude the transient homeless. Russo (1987) reports that homeless children are called "shelter kids" by their peers, that they have no sense of belonging and fail to develop long term relationships.

Recreation

McCall (1987) notes that most shelters have no recreational facilities (e.g., rec rooms, outdoor play areas) and that children are encouraged not to play with one another; shelter rules require them to be kept quiet and under direct parental supervision when outside of their sleeping quarters. This adds to the pressure and stress of the parent-child relationship, causes anger toward the parent, and further contributes to low self-esteem (Russo, 1987; McCall, 1987). In some shelters leased and operated under contract with private landlords, owners and their agents are an oppressive presence which sternly monitors and discourages children's play; vandalism, particularly by older children, is a real issue (McCall, 1987).

Community

Observers note a terrible dilemma in that both children and families are critically in need of mutual support and that feelings of community are institutionally discouraged. The temporary nature of shelter life in and of itself negates the development of bonds, even for mutual self-assistance and other support networks.

In some cases, families are "juggled" from shelter to shelter, or even feel pushed out, because municipalities are under the economic pressure of federal regulation not to allow long stays (Russo, 1987). About half of the public shelters force families back into the street every day, although they can reclaim their sleeping space at night (Waxman & Reyes, 1987).

Domestic Violence

Studies note that domestic violence increases in sheltered families, as do family break-ups (Waxman & Reyes, 1987). There was even one case reported where the noncustodial parent sought to reverse a divorce decree because of the homelessness of the other.

Child Care

Shelters require parents to be responsible for and to continually supervise their children. Even though some jurisdictions do provide child care (during the day) to *working* parents, most have inadequate or no resources for the children of unemployed homeless parents or for those working a night shift. This makes job hunting near impossible. In some cases, a sheltered child found alone immediately will be sent to foster care (McCall, 1987).

Transportation

Most sheltered parents are required to travel in order to improve their lot. In search of a job, housing, public assistance, schooling, medical attention, and even daily food, these parents receive little or no transportation aid and must bring their children with them for the lack of an alternative arrangement. This not only exacerbates the children's situations, but places an additional financial burden on parents (for children's fares) and renders it more difficult for them to accomplish their mission (Waxman & Reyes, 1987).

Social Services

Public welfare and social service agencies do not provide adequate assistance to homeless families. In fact, participation in some entitlement and other programs is prohibited by some agencies' regulations (Homeless Persons' Survival Act, 1986). Over two-thirds of the homeless parents interviewed in one study reported that their contact with public agencies was "not at all helpful" (Bassuk et al., 1986, p. 1100). Being without a fixed address can frustrate the most assertive of efforts to secure entitlements.

It is important to take note of the fact that the regulations of some entitlement programs can *force homelessness* upon families. For instance, one reason that "couch people" — those temporarily living with relatives — sometimes are asked to leave is because the host family's eligibility for public assistance, and even Food Stamps, is threatened by their presence in the household. Some agencies insist on recalculating eligibility for the host family; they want to count the income and any benefits of the temporarily housed relatives.

PROGRAM RESPONSES TO IMMEDIATE NEEDS

As should be clear, the needs of homeless children and families include and go well beyond those of even their poorest peers with permanent addresses. While some public and private programs do better than others in meeting some of those needs, none appears to offer the full range of effective services required to assure an adequate quality of life, even temporarily. Fewer programs appear to move families with children effectively and quickly out of homelessness and into a more normal life style. There appears to be even a greater paucity of government initiative to challenge the root causes of the accelerating homelessness for families and children.

In the discussion which follows, we first look at programs necessary to assist parents in addressing the problems of homeless children and families noted above. We then turn to additional areas of need and speak to policy more generally.

It is important to note the perceived tension, as often identified by public officials, between service and dependency dynamics (Alleyne, personal communication; Rowe, 1986; Pavetti, 1986). In fact, social service delivery to homeless children is purposely designed to remain within existing agency systems, rather than to be provided on site; agencies are encouraged to give the homeless priority, but discouraged from developing new programs (Pavetti, 1986).

While we recognize this dilemma, we cannot conscionably sanction a philosophy and policies which function to sustain misery, exacerbate hardship, and allow homelessness to sweep up families in an ever-growing tornado of unmet needs and despondency.

The fundamental decision which some policy makers seem to frame for themselves is a question of how much service can be provided homeless people without encouraging their dependence on shelter programs. We believe that issue needs to be reframed. The question ought to be how can homeless people, especially children and families, be served in ways which will accelerate their return to self-sufficiency and a reasonable quality of life while minimizing the continuing damage of homelessness itself.

With this position in mind, we suggest below a range of services which we believe ought to be available to homeless children and their families.

The challenge is to provide services to homeless children and families in such a way as to hasten their return to a permanent residence, and to continue to offer support and assistance for whatever period is necessary to sustain those improved circumstances. In other words, these services should truly be transitional. They should be available during and after the period of homelessness until the family is more solidly rooted in its own health and able to operate effectively in its own welfare.

Some isolated programs, such as D.C.'s CONSERVE, which already employ such an approach find it to be not only humane, but a more meaningful and effective way to tackle the multi-problem nature of homelessness (Russo, 1987). Further below we speak to post-homelessness services.

Shelter and Family Cohesion

There is an immediate and pressing need to provide adequate shelter, of reasonable quality, to homeless families and children. There is a shortage of available space for those now requesting such assistance, and they are but a minority of families and children needing it. Obviously, the first level of need is to provide shelter in ways which allow homeless families to remain together until such time as they are able to relocate to a more permanent residence.

The response of government has not been imaginative. In some jurisdictions, New York City for instance, payments are made to "welfare hotels" on the order of between $1,500 and $3,000 per month to house a single family under the most horrendous and dangerous conditions (Kurtz, 1987). The District of Columbia pays private motel owners about $90/day to house a family of three (Rowe, 1986).

Policies, on both a federal and local level, need to be established to allow such resources to be used more creatively in the provision of shelter. For instance, the aggregation of such funds could help finance the purchase and renovation of extant buildings (some of which are being "warehoused"—held out of the rental market).

Other arrangements would allow nonprofit organizations to employ these same resources more cost-effectively (than commercial landlords) in service to homeless children and their parents. Although it raises many sensitive issues, others have suggested increasing shelter capabilities by arranging the equivalent of "foster family" placements in private homes and encouraging adopt-a-family programs (Waxman & Reyes, 1987).

Schooling

Clearly, school-age children should be in school. In some cities, such as the District of Columbia, education officials do outreach to homeless families; shelter staff help to encourage attendance by assisting parents in getting children up and off to school in the morning (McCall, 1987). In localities where regulations frustrate enrollment in the school of choice (old district or shelter district), policies need to be changed. Access to school transportation, or subsidy for mass transit to/from school, needs to be provided. Ordinary entitlements to special school services and classes need to be assured (Homeless Persons' Survival Act, 1986). Clothing (and laundry facilities) adequate to school wear need to be provided (Waxman & Reyes, 1987).

School authorities ought to be encouraged to confront the issue of homelessness educationally, as well as administratively. All children (and parents) should be taught of the situation and circumstances of their (anonymous) homeless peers; empathy should be encouraged. School-based counseling should be provided both to homeless children and to other students who ridicule them.

Shelters should assure homeless children the space and quiet needed for homework and study. Shelter-based tutorial and other educational assistance programs should be provided. Some even suggest that shelters operate special schools for homeless children (Waxman & Reyes, 1987), as is being done in Salt Lake City (Henry, 1987). Outreach by public library "bookmobiles" and other organizations also would encourage and enhance education.

Psychosocial Development and Mental Health

These problems of homeless children should be recognized and operationally addressed. Diagnostic and treatment services should be made available on site at shelters by qualified personnel through public agency outreach. Therapeutic groups should be run for homeless children, parents and families; shelters ought to have the necessary space available for such programs. Referral and intensive services should be available.

Equally important are efforts to identify those dynamics which contribute to the onset or exacerbation of these problems. Care should be taken to help homeless parents to develop the skills necessary to support their children during such difficult times. Shelter life needs to be examined and understood as a culture, and its negative impact on families moderated through thoughtful intervention. Enrichment and other compensatory programs are needed to facilitate children's development. Some recommend special Head-Start programs for sheltered children (Waxman & Reyes, 1987).

Physical Health

Adequate hygiene needs to be promoted and maintained in sheltered families; necessary sanitary facilities must be provided. Reasonable health care for minor illnesses and ailments ought to be made available by visiting medical personnel and access to clinics and hospitals ought to be facilitated when needed.

Substance abuse programs need to be available and open to homeless parents and youth. Some existing programs would demand little in new resources. Many require significant commitments by participants; shelter staff should support parents and children in beginning and maintaining involvement.

Nutrition

Care needs to be taken to assure adequate diet for homeless children and their parents. When shelters do not provide prepared food through a cafeteria or other arrangement, individual families need assistance in the purchase and preparation of meals. Appropriate facilities need to be provided. Arrangements need to be made for food stamps, acquisition of surplus food, and/or feeding by other nearby and accessible programs. One recommendation is to relax requirements for eligibility and to allow the use of food stamps at shelter feeding programs (Homeless Persons' Survival Act, 1986). Particular attention needs to be paid to the dietary needs of infants and expectant mothers.

Infants

Homeless families with infants have special needs which must be accommodated to avoid permanent damage to the very young. Infant care and stimulation programs ought to be available and special shelters ought to house them and their parents. Close attention ought to be paid to monitoring infant development and necessary remedial services ought to be provided on site. Parenting an infant is sometimes difficult under ordinary circumstances and may be horrendous for the homeless; respite and support ought to be available to the parents of very young children.

Peer Relationships

Friendship among homeless children, and between them and their peers with permanent residences, ought to be facilitated. Through peer-support groups, open discussions and other methods, homeless children should be helped to identify problems they are experiencing with others of their age.

Recreation

Shelters should assure children use of indoor and outdoor recreation facilities and encourage play. Where necessary, cooperative or staffed arrangements for adult supervision should be facilitated. Russo (1987) even suggests that organized adult recreation (such as softball teams) would help alleviate some parental depression and lethargy.

Some cities, such as the District of Columbia, have provided access and transportation to summer day camp programs (McCall, 1987), but year-round resources are missing in most localities. Efforts should be made to incorporate homeless children in recreational programs available in shelter neighborhoods, both from public and private agencies, encouraging their integration with their peers. After-school programs should be made available at shelters and/or in public schools for homeless children.

Community

Self-help and peer-support networks among homeless families should be facilitated by shelter staff. Efforts should be made to assist these families to build (or recreate) the kinds of support networks necessary to maintain life free of dependency on public resources. Extended networks, including some that draw on volunteers from more solidly grounded families, ought to be created in lieu of extended biological families. Homeless children and parents should be encouraged to participate in local organizations and community life (while recognizing and helping them overcome barriers to such activity).

Staff should help stable families to form babysitting and child care cooperatives and other social organizations such as welcoming committees for incoming parents and their children. Community celebrations for exiting families would be a very positive way to reinforce hope in those who remain. Such rites of passage also would allow trained clinical staff to help exiting and remaining children with transitions and feelings of separation and loss.

Domestic Violence

Clearly domestic violence can never be tolerated and the staff of shelters should be trained in its identification and remediation. Incoming parents should receive an orientation to shelter life and be given assistance in anticipating and dealing with the likely strains on the family. Family and spousal counseling should be available in shelters. Emphasis should be placed on prevention of spousal and/

or child abuse and immediate response to its occurrence. Special family-oriented day programs have been recommended (Waxman & Reyes, 1987).

Child Care

One observer reports that the paucity of child care is a major contributor to homelessness because it both causes unemployment and restricts employability (Alleyne, personal communication, 1987). Clearly, no other service beyond shelter itself is as essential to a homeless parent's efforts to remedy the situation than is child care. The difficulty of a homeless parent needing to take a child along on an employment search or interview, a negotiation with a potential landlord, etc., should be clear. The possibility of holding a job, especially one on the night shift, becomes infinitesimally small for a homeless parent without child care resources. Such services must be made available to homeless families, preferably on site at shelters.

Transportation

The mobility of homeless parents and children is requisite to their efforts to maintain themselves and improve their lives. Beyond getting to and from schools, job interviews, housing searches, income maintenance and other services, all require movement around town. Subsidies for mass transit are necessary and small group transport services, via a van for instance, would greatly facilitate the accomplishment of these necessary tasks. If a whole day and significant fare is required to get to and from an appointment with an employment counselor, for instance, homelessness will not quickly be corrected. The hassle of daily life needs to be minimized for a homeless parent trying to keep a family together.

Social Services

Federal and local policies which penalize homelessness by restricting access to entitlements (such as AFDC, Social Security, Food Stamps, etc.) and other social service programs need to be modified immediately (Homeless Persons' Survival Act, 1986;

Melnick & Williams, 1987). Not to do so is patently absurd and incredibly inhumane.

Public and private agency personnel need to be sensitized to the circumstances of homeless parents and children, and practices which further victimize those requiring service must be quashed. Priority needs to be given families without a home in any effort which might alleviate their horrendous conditions and facilitate a return to a more normal life.

Help in the form of technical assistance and advocacy needs to be given homeless families, it is regrettable to say, in dealing with the very agencies and personnel who are supposed to be responsive to them. One suggestion offered is to move toward a "case management" approach to dealing with the multiple problems of homeless families (Waxman & Reyes, 1987; Homeless Persons' Survival Act, 1986).

PROGRAM RESPONSES TO ADDITIONAL NEEDS

Beyond these efforts, there is a range of additional services which homeless children and their parents require if they are to be supported in improving on their present situation. These are more directly related to the circumstances which led to their homelessness than are many of the other areas discussed above.

Housing Assistance

The obvious cause of homelessness is the paucity of affordable housing. While the long-range nature of this problem is discussed below, its immediate implications must be addressed for homeless families. Assistance needs to be provided in helping them to find and secure a permanent residence.

Families need housing counseling services to help them identify appropriate dwellings and they need to be given assistance (perhaps even through legislation) in receiving priority consideration as tenants. They need coaching and support, even advocacy, in dealing with prospective landlords. They need financial assistance adequate to security deposit and rent guarantee demands (Waxman & Reyes, 1987).

It should be noted that even where some such assistance is available to homeless families, the realities of the rental housing market are such as to render them highly ineffective. This is addressed below.

Employment

Beyond available units, affordable housing implies the family's ability to pay rent regularly and on a continuing basis. This means that they need reasonable levels of income.

Job training, employment search, and job retention skills are needed by the parents of homeless children, and by some of the older youth themselves. One recommendation is that homelessness alone ought to qualify someone for entry into job training programs (Homeless Persons' Survival Act, 1986). Whatever the services, it is clear that unless these parents are assisted in finding, qualifying for, and keeping reasonable employment, they and their children will continue to be among the homeless.

It needs to be remembered that many of the homeless already are employed. At current minimum wage levels, a family of four with both parents working (one full-time and one half-time) still falls well below the established poverty line. Federal economic policy is creating large number of working, and increasingly homeless, poor families.

Legal Issues

Problems seem to compound one another and it is not rare that a family down on its luck finds itself somehow involved in the legal system. Homeless families are not unique in this regard; they require legal services, counseling and advocacy, as well as other related support services (Waxman & Reyes, 1987).

Post-Homelessness Services

While we might have made the reader despair that homeless families ever find permanent residence, such is not the case. However, when they do succeed in locating and obtaining housing, they need support to maintain and increase their self-reliance.

Beyond the continuation of many of the kinds of services noted above, such families should have available additional training in budgeting and financial management, time management, stress management and conflict resolution, and should generally be able to draw on a variety of support networks and crisis-intervention resources. McCall (1987) noted that transitional and continued service is essential to break the disheartening pattern which she observes of large numbers of homeless families becoming "repeaters" — those who manage to leave shelters for a more normal life and who soon find themselves back on the street again.

Root Cause: Affordable Housing

As has been noted over and over again by experts across the nation, the root cause of homelessness is the paucity of affordable housing. Most alarmingly, this situation grows worse steadily.

In congressional testimony reporting on a national survey, Raymond Flynn (1987), Chair of the United States Conference of Mayor's Task Force on Hunger and Homelessness, noted that the demand for low-income housing increased last year by 40%, that the average wait for assisted housing is 18 months (although two-thirds of the surveyed cities are facing such a level of demand that they have felt forced to close their waiting lists), and that over the past five years the stock of available low and moderate income housing *decreased or did not grow* in over 70% of the surveyed cities.

As mentioned above, a study done by Phillip Clay at the Massachusetts Institute of Technology on behalf of the Neighborhood Reinvestment Corporation (cited in Jordan, 1987) found that 18.7 million U.S. residents will be homeless (or very nearly homeless) within 16 years if these trends remain unchecked. There appears to be not even the faintest hope that our society will be able to provide them with the shelter and services called for above.

It is only a major rethinking of public policy that can change the future foretold by these projections. Our nation cannot deal with the coming specter of millions upon millions of homeless children unless we change government housing policies at the federal level.

During the past five years under the Reagan administration, federal housing assistance was *cut by over 75%* (Flynn, 1987). There can be no better illustration of the fact that current government policy is putting increasingly large numbers of children and their parents into the streets. We contend that these disastrous and destructive policies must be changed.

There are myriad legislative efforts underway to ameliorate this horror; many were cited by Flynn (1987) in his testimony. Most are failing to gain the administrative and congressional support necessary to their enactment. Thus, more important than the specifics of any number of possible approaches is the question of the will and commitment of our nation.

Our choices are simple: we can fret about increasing the dependency of the homeless while millions more are created, or we can demand resolute action to change our society, to bring our children home.

REFERENCES

Alleyne, S. (1987, May) *Development of a needs assessment instrument and pilot study of homeless families in the District of Columbia*. Unpublished masters thesis, National Catholic School of Social Services, Catholic University of America, Washington, D.C.

Associated Press. (1987, October 17). Welfare cuts rescinded for charity takers. *The Washington Post*, p. A11.

Bassuk, E.L., Rubin, L., & Lauriat, A.S. (1986, September). Characteristics of sheltered homeless families. *American Journal of Public Health, 76*(9), 1097-1101.

Center for Law and Education (1987, April 21). *Education problems of homeless children and suggested legislative language changes*. Washington.

Collier, M. (1986, December 8). Quick plunge from the suburbs to the shelters. *The Oakland Tribune*, pp. A1-A2.

Dobbin, M. (1987, August 3). The children of the homeless. *U.S. News and World Report*, pp. 19-21.

Flynn, R.L. (1987, February 4). *Testimony before the subcommittee on housing and community development; committee on banking, finance and urban affairs; U.S. House of Representatives*. Washington: United States Conference of Mayors.

Haddock, V. (1986, December 11). Homeless children increasing. *The Oakland Tribune*, pp. A1-A2.

Henry, N. (1987, June 21). A shelter for learning. *The Washington Post*, pp. A1, A16-A17.

Homeless Persons' Survival Act of 1986. Washington: U.S. House of Representatives.

Jordan, M. (1987, June 3). 18 million homeless seen by 2003. *The Washington Post*, p. A8.

Kurtz, H. (1987, September 15). Welfare hotel occupants at eye of political storm in New York. *The Washington Post*, p. A3.

Lane, J.B., & Depp, F.C. (1987). *Sheltered homeless in the nation's capital: a comparison study of characteristics, needs and services for Washington, D.C. homeless single adults and families* (Report to D.C. Commission on Homelessness, Department of Human Services). Washington: Howard University Department of Occupational Therapy.

Martin, M. (1987, September). Homeless families. In M. Martin (Chair) *Homeless Families*. Annual Meeting of the Profession, National Association of Social Workers, New Orleans.

Maza, P.L., & Hall, J.A. (1986). *Study of homeless children and families, preliminary findings*. Washington: Travelers Aid International and Child Welfare League of America.

Melnick, V.L., & Williams, C.S. (1987, May). *Children and families without homes: observations from thirty case studies*. Washington: University of the District of Columbia, Center for Applied Research and Urban Policy.

Reyes, L.M., & Waxman, L.D. (1986, December). *The continued growth of hunger, homelessness and poverty in America's cities: 1986*. Washington: United States Conference of Mayors.

Rivlin, L.G. (1986, Spring). A new look at the homeless. *Social Policy*, *16*(4), 3-10.

Robinson, F.G. (1985, November). *Homeless people in the nation's capital* (D.C. Homelessness Study No. 1). Washington: University of the District of Columbia, Center for Applied Research and Urban Policy.

Rowe, A. (1986, December). *Comprehensive plan for homeless families*. Washington: Commission on Social Services, Department of Human Resources, District of Columbia Government.

Russell, Seabook, Father McKenna Center and National Coalition for the Homeless v. Barry, Hawkins and Bowen, No. 87-2072, DC (1987).

Waxman, L.D., & Reyes, L.M. (1987, May). *A status report on homeless families in America's cities*. Washington: United States Conference of Mayors.

Whitman, D., & Bosc, M. (1987, August 3). The coming of the couch people. *U.S. News and World Report*, pp. 19-21.

Winerip, M. (1987, October 6). Our towns: the education of Des Paganelli: who will do it? *The New York Times*, p. B1

Homeless Women and Children:
The Question of Poverty

Stanley F. Battle, PhD

ABSTRACT. Many changes have occurred in this country that influence personalities, values, and institutions which bring about a marked change in the functioning of society as a whole. These changes have been most dramatic within the institution of the family where they have had a most telling effect on personal lives. Poverty as an independent factor is arguably the single most important determinant of health status in the United States. Low birth weight, malnutrition and housing are a few examples of how poverty can affect the lives of family members. This chapter will address poverty in the context of homeless women and children and how they are influenced based on our national agenda. Government programs will be explored to highlight how the culture of poverty is used as a defense mechanism to explain poverty and homelessness.

Much of our attention these days is centered on changes that are critical in the labor market and what this nation will look like in the year 2000. We are presently debating what roles the public and private sectors will play in regard to our economic position internationally while we neglect social conditions which have a profound effect on the country. It is difficult to measure social stability and equality, but we have a crisis in this country that greatly affects

Stanley F. Battle, received his MSW degree from the University of Connecticut School of Social Work in 1975 and his MPH in 1979 and PhD in 1980 from the University of Pittsburgh Schools of Public Health and Social Work. Presently, Dr. Battle is Associate Professor of Welfare Policy and Health at the University of Connecticut School of Social Work. Dr. Battle is Coordinator of the Black Experience Sequence/Institute. He serves as consultant to several local, state and federal programs. His research focus is on mental health issues affecting minorities with a special interest in Black adolescent males.

111

women and children. Forty percent of white children live in poverty as opposed to 60% of Black children. The fastest growing poverty group in the U.S. are women and children, and they constitute the new wave of homeless persons today. In Chicago, there are an estimated 25,000 homeless persons and 2,500 available beds; Boston has between 14,000-17,000 homeless persons, of whom many are intact families (husband, wife, and children). Homelessness has affected people who have worked their entire lives, for example, auto and steel employees. Detroit mayor Coleman Young asked the governor to declare his city a disaster area. Poverty as an independent factor is arguably the single most important determinant of health status in the United States. Low birth weight, malnutrition and housing are a few examples of how poverty can affect the lives of family members. One of the most profound experiences of the poor is when they are forced out of their homes and communities, and thus lose their identity and recognition. Homeless people are totally alone in their experiences and much of their frustration is directed toward family members. Feelings of guilt, rage, and denial are common. This chapter will address poverty in the context of homeless women and children.

WOMEN IN THE WORKFORCE

Thirty years ago, women were less than one-third of the labor force. In 1986, 44% of the labor force was female and 50% of all women worked outside of the home. By the year 2000, 47% of the total workforce will be female and 60% of all women will work outside of the home. Projections for 1985-1995 in regard to the welfare system and how women and children will be treated are open to speculation. More than half (62%) of all women with children under 18 are employed; more than half (54%) of all women with children under 6 are in the labor force. Almost half of all married mothers with infants age 1 or younger are either working or looking for work (Battle, 1986).

More women are entering the labor force, but they do not receive their fair share in wages. Women earn 40 cents less on the dollar than men. Boston, Massachusetts is one of the most progressive areas in the U.S., but poverty and unemployment are not strangers to Boston. Consider the following example. Many of our urban areas exemplify *A Tale of Two Cities*. In Boston, the city's unemployment rate is one of the lowest in the nation, while its poverty rate is one of the highest. The percentage of Bostonians living below the federal poverty line, which the U.S. Census Bureau determines as an income which is less than $10,609 for family of four, increased from 16% in 1970 to 20% in 1980, five percent higher than the national average. The Boston Redevelopment Association estimates that in five years, 23% of the populations, or nearly one in every four Boston residents, will be impoverished (Battle, 1986).

Women frequently work for minimum wage, thus boosting the poverty rates, and many end up on welfare because there are no other appropriate options. In real dollars, the buying power of checks from Aid to Families with Dependent Children (AFDC) decreased by 33% from 1978-1983. Also, in real dollars, compared to the average U.S. wage, the minimum wage is at its lowest level in half a century. If a person making minimum wage ($3.35 an hour) were to work full time, 40 hours per week, 52 weeks a year, he or she would earn, before taxes, $7200.00 This is more than $3,000 under the poverty level for a family of four. Many have argued that these three factors have led to the deterioration of the family (Battle, 1986).

The group of people who are directly affected by income factors are children. Poverty among children is alarming, but its ramifications appear to be silent. In 1985, one of every four children under 17 lived in poverty. A trend of increasing numbers of children in poverty has been described by the Census Bureau since 1973, with the largest increase since 1980. Half of the increases in poverty among families with children between 1981-1985 were due to the declining impact of government assistance programs in moving families from poverty. In 1985, only one family out of every nine with children was removed from poverty by these programs, compared to one family out of five in 1979 (Report Policy Priorities, 1986). For instance, program benefits are frequently reduced and medical coverage denied to many working poor, which penalizes people who work for low wages. Programs developed to correct economic fluctuations of the poor, such as Aid to Families with Dependent Children (AFDC) and food stamps do not provide adequate assistance and in many respects maintain poor families below the poverty line and induce dependency on the welfare system (The Physician Report, 1985).

A variety of factors may push a family into homelessness: the loss of the primary breadwinner who did not have health insurance, unemployment or the loss of permanent shelter. In the final analysis, the mother is generally left with the responsibility of caring for the children. The policies of various government administrations have not fully addressed the needs of the poor and homeless.

GOVERNMENT PROGRAMS

In January 1982, President Reagan cited some $44 billion in cuts already obtained in social programs, and announced his intention to continue this trend with another $63 billion in savings over the next several years. Reflected in these figures was the President's approach to dealing with the system in which "available resources are going not to the greedy" (Palmer & Sawhill, 1982). While the Reagan Administration has been ferreting out the "greedy" and acting on its belief that most individuals can adequately fend for themselves in a free market economy, many social policies have been neglected.

Some experts argue that poverty is caused by deviance of the lower class. In order to correct this flaw, programs would be developed to alter the deviant individual or subculture. We have not developed an intellectual theory base to explain homelessness.

Particular trends in American society reflect greater adherence to one theory or conceptual model to address the needs of the poor. Prior to the Great Depression, the federal government played a limited role in addressing the needs of the poor. Private organizations such as churches and local community groups as well as large extended families took the responsibility of caring for the worthy poor. Those individuals who were considered the destitute and unworthy poor were removed from society and sent to alms houses.

The concept of "undeserving" poor during the period prior to the 1930s parallels what later became the culture of poverty view. From this earlier perception of the unworthy poor evolved the culture of poverty which in addition to attributing deviant behavior also held that individual rehabilitation was necessary to eliminate economic deprivation.

The Great Depression forced American society to re-examine the belief in the "work ethic" when even hard workers were subject to economic disaster. Workers were vulnerable to social and economic factors which ran contrary to the belief that poverty, for the most part, was an affliction of those who did not work hard. The basic tenets of the work ethic could neither explain nor alleviate the massive unemployment and poverty which swept through the nation and affected workers.

The concept of New Deal programs was revolutionary in that for the first time in American history the federal government intervened in the economic protection of individual Americans, heretofore a private issue. Programs initiated by the Roosevelt Administration were designed to guard against the kind of fluctuation in the national economy which had precipitated disaster during the Great Depression. New Deal policies stressed work for the worthy poor and sought to maintain economic independence and morale, as well as benefits to the elderly, a minimum wage and unemployment insurance. The anti-poverty program instituted by the New Deal carried the message that the victims were not responsible for the failure of the economy and, moreover, the government would rescue them from the poverty that resulted.

The most recent public effort to eradicate poverty in the U.S.; second in scope only to the New Deal was the War on Poverty during the Kennedy and Johnson Administrations of the 1960s. While the New Deal addressed eliminating poverty through economic mechanisms, the War on Poverty initially attempted to get at the causes of poverty which were seen as resulting from a lack of political and decision-making power. Programs developed during the 1960s were considered revolutionary in that never before in American history had an attempt been made to alter the social structure in order to eliminate poverty. Political leadership of the time portrayed the War on Poverty as a major assault on power and opportunity structures in America.

The War on Poverty efforts initially dealt with providing access to various socio-economic opportunities for the poor. The Economic Act of 1964 (EOA) opened the door to participation of the poor in the social structure by fostering their involvement. Acclaimed as the "total war on poverty," the stated aims of the Economic Opportunity Act were to eliminate poverty and to restructure the role of the poor in society by involving them in program design and administration (Levitan, 1969). These goals would be achieved through Community Action Programs (CAPs) which called for "maximum feasible participation" of residents of the poor community in program development and administration. It is important to understand that while the EOA encouraged direct involvement of the poor themselves in local policy making and planning boards, local government and mayors criticized CAPs for changing the locus of decision-making control.

The War on Poverty was a period racked with struggles and ideological differences. This period occurred during the same period, and in many respects as a result of the Civil Rights Movement. Blacks were disproportionately represented among people living in poverty and were subject to barriers in access to opportunity in the social and economic structure. A National Advisory Committee on Civil Disorder was set up to study the conditions of Black America. The Kerner Commission report cited the failure of the dominant social structure to eradicate poverty and to end racial discrimination. It documented the prohibition of blacks from participation in dominant white society as the cause of high unemployment, inadequate housing, crime and insecurity, poor health and sanitation conditions, and exploitation of consumers. Indeed the racism experienced by blacks may explain perceived differences in chances for success between blacks and whites.

The War on Poverty achieved some success in reducing poverty but the battles implemented were not based on its original ideals. In response to opposition to proposed changes in the social structure, the emphasis of the War on Poverty largely shifted to programs designed to change the poor. Staffing of Community Action Programs which had so strongly advocated direct participation of the local poor in decisions regarding their own welfare, mainly consisted of non-poor individuals, including poverty consultants and advocacy groups, in competition for the poverty grants. Improvements in advocacy for the poor were suggested which would minimally improve the condition of the poor while maintaining the existing social power structure.

The failure of the War on Poverty to remove barriers in access to power and opportunity led some policy makers away from attempts to alter the power structure in America. In 1969, Moynihan, then Nixon's Social Policy Advisor advocated a guaranteed annual income program to increase access to resources and economic opportunity for the poor. The "Family Action Plan" (FAP) considered by the Nixon Administration would guarantee an annual income to all American citizens in order to mitigate inefficiencies within the existing welfare system (The President's Commission, 1970). The FAP idea was similar to a negative income level, the government pays citizens in proportion to their lack of income, rather than the progressive income tax in which citizens pay the government in proportion to their income.

Political difficulties with the proposal led to its defeat. The plan required employment as a condition to receive assistance. There were two problems inherent in requiring employment. First, earning a wage plus an additional guaranteed income could deny some families eligibility for other assistance programs such as Medicaid and Food Stamps. For those families it would make more sense not to work. Second, people would not work if there were no jobs. In addition, welfare assistance had been provided by states at different benefit levels. In states with high benefit levels, the poor were worse off, in states with low benefits, the FAP would provide a large increase and would be viewed as politically unacceptable.

Although policies during the 1960s did not totally eradicate poverty in the U.S., the number of people living in poverty was reduced due to far-reaching welfare reforms and increased employment opportunities. But the lack of support for the policies aimed at changing the social structure, to transfer power, and increase opportunity among the poor led to the development of programs to alter behavior and the value systems of the poor.

The Reagan plan is designed to address the needs of the poor through indirect means. The plan states that stimulating economic growth through minimally regulated private enterprise would benefit all, even the poor. The Administration asserts that government intervention would hamper this economic revitalization process. Our present Administration reverts back to ideological approaches prior to the Great Depression, which stressed the value of the work ethic. Within this system, there are winners and losers.

The rate of poverty through tax programs has actually worsened the economic plight of poor families. Between 1978 (Carter Administration) and 1984 (Reagan Administration) the income tax burden on families of four with poverty level income rose 400% in dollar amount and rose 250% in percentage of income. Poor families paid 4% of their income in taxes in 1978; in 1984 they paid 10.1%. Between 1983 and 1985 income was actually transferred from poor to wealthy families. The combined effect of tax policies during those three years was to transfer $23.1 billion from poor families with annual incomes of $10,000 or less, and to give an additional $34.9 billion to families with annual incomes of over $80,000 (Task Force on Hunger, 1985).

In effect, what we have seen is a return to the traditional thinking of the early 20th century, or earlier. The emergence of the Poor Law and the Progressive Era reflect much of our present-day understanding of the poor. But how do the homeless families fit into the scheme?

THE HOMELESS POPULATION

A growing proportion of the homeless are families that are burned out, evicted or have left their apartments because of intolerable physical or safety conditions. These families cannot find new housing, partly because of the escalating rents and partly because of gentrification of their old neighborhoods. They are forced to double or triple up with relatives or friends in already overcrowded quarters. As a last resort, they are forced to move into welfare hotels or shelters. Except for their need for permanent shelter, their most urgent requirement is medical care. From a need and prevention point of view the homeless are a critical public health risk. Public shelters are a breeding ground for tuberculosis, respiratory disease, and parasitic diseases. The homeless have six times the rate of neurological disease, five times the kidney and liver disease, and thirty times the number of skin ulcers and lesions than the rest of the population (Mailick, 1985).

Many of the homeless families frequently have existing chronic health problems and congregate living adds to the risk of acute illness. Some families have children who are acutely ill and denied access to temporary housing shelters because of the fear of spreading the illness. Many families sleep in parking lots, on the floor in community centers, or they ride the subway trains all night. Frequently, city and county hospitals—like Boston City and Cook County in Chicago—are the only hospitals willing to treat this population. Hospitalization is generally short term; consequently there is little time available to develop treatment plans to meet survival needs.

One of the most dramatic changes in the composition of the homeless is the large increase in homeless families (Acre & Vergare, 1984; HUD, 1984). In 1986, an increase in homeless families with children was reported by 80% of 25 cities surveyed in the U.S. (Reyes & Waxman, 1986). The demand for shelters has increased by over 20% in large urban settings. The 1985 Massachusetts Report on Homelessness estimated that 75% of the homeless are families (Homeless Families, 1987). The number of families that are "near homeless" has increased dramatically from 1980-1986.

Homeless Families

Massachusetts is considered one of the most progressive states in the country and it has one of the lowest unemployment rates as well. But, every day in Massachusetts between 200 and 500 families are housed in shelters, and between 400 and 500 families are supported in hotels and motels (Bassuk, Rubin & Lauriat, 1986). Estimates of homeless families statewide, as previously indicated in the 1985 Massachusetts Report on Homelessness, is 75%. On a national level, the average rate of homeless families with children is between 21% and 28%. The figures are somewhat misleading. Many women with children who are not citizens of this country are not counted.

Historically, there have been more men among the homeless than women. Although the numbers of women have increased, men still comprise a majority of the population. Nationwide, single men make up 66% of the homeless, single women 13%, and families 21% (HUD, 1984). Among homeless adult family members, a 1985 Boston study showed that 90.1% of the homeless families are female-headed, 8.5% couple-headed, and 1.4% male-headed (HUD, 1984; *Boston's Homeless*, 1986). This is the reverse of the gender distribution among homeless individuals. Throughout the state, approximately 80% of homeless families are headed by female single parents. The growing number of female-headed homeless families continues to grow and we have not developed any real policy to address the needs of this population. Can homelessness be explained as a denial of economic resources or is it an outgrowth effect of our economic system?

Dysfunctional Economic Structure

The dysfunctional economic system model holds that poverty is caused by uncontrolled changes in the national economy, resulting in distress for the most vulnerable. In this view, the lower class is cut off from economic opportunity available to other Americans by changes in the national economy. Worthiness in the United States is based on the ability to compete. All decent or worthy people work hard and are able to care for themselves and their families as a result. Conversely, those who are unemployed or have inadequate income come under the close scrutiny of the federal government. Poor people are viewed as unworthy by many and suffer economic neglect at the hand of the federal government.

Historically, the culture of poverty advanced in American sociology and social theory in the 1940s, 1950s and the early 1960s focused on this purported social deviance of the poor to explain social and economic inequality (blaming the victim). The behavioral norms of the poor were viewed as deviant from the norms of mainstream American society and as such, formed a social subculture. Moreover, the behavior of the subculture was viewed as a determinant of its low economic status. For instance, according to the Urban Institute, during the recession of the late 1970s and the early 1980s income inequality increased. Disposable income among the most wealthy Americans increased by 8.4%, while disposable income among the poorest fell by 7.6% (Physician Task Force on Hunger, 1985). Based on this theory, proponents feel that learning to control the economy will help prevent recession and eliminate poverty in the nation.

When we consider the plight of the homeless, poverty and its results are viewed as deviant. The culture of poverty has been the accepted concept used to explain homelessness. Poor people, it is held, adopt maladaptive values and deviant behaviors which determine and maintain their low economic status. In this view, the value system and behavior of the poor represents a deviant "subculture" which does not adhere to the norms and goals of the larger American society. As a result, poverty and homelessness results from character flaws and social deviance.

The basis for this thinking is the Elizabethan Poor Laws of 1601, still greatly reflected in the Protestant work ethic in America. The poor laws created two categories of impoverished citizens. The worthy poor were widows, orphans, the elderly, and the disabled. They were viewed as members of the larger society whose external misfortunes had determined their poverty. They were deserving of care from the community. The unworthy were largely unemployed heads of households and unmarried males who were seen as a separate group. Their ablebodiness, along with their poverty was ample demonstration of their deviance and lack of virtue. The homeless are a combination of the two; they reflect our fears, realizations and denial.

The Elizabethan Poor Laws recognized children as worthy of care, but throughout history children had been exploited and misunderstood. Homelessness affects children in a very real sense; some are totally helpless while others select the street as an option to intolerable living conditions at home.

Case Example: Homeless Children

Homeless youth are a sub-population of runaway youths who are under the age of eighteen. Homeless youth can be described in two groups: (1) children who live with their parents and become victims because parent(s) lose their jobs; and (2) children who become homeless because they run away from home. Only 50% of runaway youths will eventually return home or find a permanent placement (Chelimsky, 1982).

The Runaway and Homeless Youth Act was passed in 1974 to provide grants and technical assistance to agencies to develop and support community-based programs. The Act has resulted in service to only about 6% of the runaway population (Chelimsky, 1982).

A group that needs careful consideration when we look at homeless children are adolescent parents. Possibly the most important social problem challenging the family today is the rate of adolescent pregnancy and its aftermath.

The phenomenon of unprecedented rates of adolescent pregnancy and childbearing in the 1970s, often referred to in crisis terms as an "epidemic" appears to be receding in the 1980s. By 1982, fertility rates for teenagers had declined. Yet these birth rates, especially for adolescents, are still disturbingly high. They are not only among the highest levels ever observed for the United States, but they are among the highest in the Western industrial world.

While the number of births to teenagers (656,000 in 1970, 562,000 in 1980, and 537,024 in 1981) gives us the dimensions of the problem, these aggregate numbers mask the distinct differences among age groups within the adolescent populations (Guttmacher, 1981).

While the uneven rates of decline in birth rates within the adolescent cohort is noteworthy, the dramatic story of the last two decades is the sharp rise of teen births that are out-of-wedlock. In 1970, nearly 70% of all teen births were legitimated by marriage. In 1980, this figure dropped to 52%. The number of out-of-wedlock births to women under 20 years of age tripled between 1960 and 1981. Almost 50% of all births to women under age 19 are out-of-wedlock (Guttmacher, 1981).

The phenomenon of out-of-wedlock births is reinforced with the recognition that the number of births to married women has declined so that a higher proportion of children are now "illegitimate." Indeed, while the number of children living with a divorced mother more than doubled between 1970 and 1982, the overall number of children living with an unmarried mother increased by a factor of more than five (Battle, 1986).

While we are unable to account with specificity for the rise, and fall of out-of-wedlock rates by age and race, it is perhaps reasonable to assume that for young black teenage women, the concerted efforts through various community programs have produced a downward trend. The upward trend for white females is accounted for perhaps by an increase in sexual activity.

While the rate of out-of-wedlock births is very high in this country, significant variation by age and race should be noted. Younger age groups within the cohort show the least decline. Moreover, looking at the racial factor, one notes that the rate is increasing for young white women and decreasing slightly for young black women. However, this should not obscure the fact that very high rates of out-of-wedlock births exist, especially for large urban areas.

Whether or not the high proportion of out-of-wedlock births signals the beginning of a family formation that will be accepted without societal stigma remains to be seen. While societal attitudes of acceptance may be more the rule, the poverty status of illegitimate children persists. Indeed, one of the most powerful predictors of a child's destiny is the family structure into which it is born. To be born to an unmarried mother places the child at the highest risk for poverty. Among all single parents (separated, divorced, widowed and unmarried), it is the children of unmarried mothers who suffer the greatest economic deprivation, and by virtue of their status, they are considered useless in society.

In many respects, changes in the AFDC program (Aid to Families with Dependent Children) have caused an estimated 400,000 to 500,000 families (about 11%-14% of the total case-load) to lose their AFDC eligibility; most of these families also lost their Medicaid benefits. Because of changes in government programs the poor and near poor can be pushed into homelessness. Some of these people have full time jobs (Palmer & Sawhill, 1982). Additionally, state-established income eligibility levels have been lowered, disqualifying millions of people whose incomes fall below the poverty line, yet exceed the low Medicaid income standards (Butler, 1985). To qualify for Medicaid, a family of four must have an income of less than $5,340. Further compounding an already enormous problem, all measures of the poverty rate rose rapidly starting in 1980 after two decades of rapid decline in that rate. By the end of 1982, the official rate was nearly as high as the beginning of the War on Poverty in 1965.

Young adolescent mothers face the dilemma of selecting how they will support their children and where to place priorities. In 1986, the poverty level threshold was approximately $5,360 for a single individual, and $10,987 for a family of four. People represented by these statistics are forced to make decisions between housing and adequate health care because of limited resources. These decisions are difficult for adults, but a sixteen-year old who is in an independent living situation is really at high risk and may make the wrong decision. Homelessness for this population is not absolute; but more single adolescent mothers (aged 17-25) are utilizing shelters, particularly in urban centers, than ever before.

Where Do We Go from Here?

Several attempts have been made throughout American history to eliminate poverty, yet it still persists. Although America is the wealthiest nation on earth, nearly 14% of its people continue to live in poverty. Anti-poverty policies have been designed to alleviate poverty by variously changing the economic structure, the social order, or even the poor themselves. But actual programs implemented by the government to reduce poverty have had varying degrees of success.

The success or failure of public policy to alleviate poverty has been strongly influenced by socio-political factors in the nation at different points in our history. FDR's New Deal policies were implemented at a time in American history when the socioeconomic structure was in a state of turmoil. New Deal programs were highly successful in part because they received widespread support. America needed swift and far-reaching change and the New Deal promised to bring prosperity back to Americans. But attempts to reduce poverty through public policy were not always met with public enthusiasm. Programs proposed as part of the War on Poverty, for example, threatened the existing power structure in American society. Due to conflict between the stated intent of public policy and the opposition to such policy by powerful interests, programs frequently became weakened versions of great intentions.

RECOMMENDATIONS AND CONCLUSIONS

At every point in the nation's history, the United States has confronted a dilemma over whether to give greater priority to reducing the economic insecurity and poverty of single parent families or reduce the number of these families and the degree of dependence on government. The number of homeless families, single or intact, continues to expand. By now many of us have had some contact with the homeless. In our large urban cities the problem has taken on new meaning, because "they" do not all fit the common stereotype of being "bums"; they are also women, children, and intact families.

Homelessness can be divided into three categories: chronic, episodic, and situational. Chronic homeless persons generally live on the street for long periods of time. Episodic homeless persons alternate between living on the street and a temporary residence. The situational homeless are generally going through some type of acute personal crisis. Generally, situational homelessness applies to homeless families, battered women and runaway youth, while adults make up the majority of chronic and episodic homeless. Homeless women and children reflect a struggle with our overall philosophy of providing services to the worthy!

Through history, we have evidence of industrial poverty in an agrarian society, 1865-1890; the impact of the urban poor during the progressive era, 1890-1920; the Great Depression, 1930-1940; and the influence of Moynihan, Harrington, and Grier and Cobbs, 1940 to the present to guide us. Homelessness is not new, but we have given it more attention because working and middle class people have become victims.

It would be courageous and controversial if state legislatures decided to provide universal care to the homeless. It is an unlikely outcome to the current political process. However, the American public cannot help but give consideration to a major intervention plan for the poor and homeless.

There are always problems with universal plans, but the following should be considered.

1. Universal access to comprehensive health services can be achieved without runaway costs. It costs $55,000 (average cost per year) to provide services to an infant who is born prematurely in the United States.
2. States need greater flexibility with federal government support to determine priorities so that regional needs can be satisfied.

3. Initiatives in the delivery of health care services can begin at the local level.

The present-day leadership has already cut benefits to an estimated 400,000 to 500,000 AFDC families and nearly one million potential food stamp beneficiaries, whereas outlays on defense have nearly doubled, from $157 billion in 1981 to $173.4 billion in 1986. Our urban centers are becoming wastelands with a variety of problems, and homelessness is just one. In the final analysis, we are all at risk. Services should be provided because to do so is right and decent.

REFERENCES

Acre, A.A., & Veragre, M.J. (1984). Identifying and Characterizing the Mentally Ill Among the Homeless. H.R. Lamb (Ed.), *The Homeless Mentally Ill: A Task Force Report of the American Psychiatric Association*.

Boston's Homeless — Taking The Next Step (1986). Boston Emergency Shelter Commission and the Planning Corporation.

Bassuk, E.L., Rubin, L., & Lauriat, A.S. (1986). Characteristics of Sheltered Homeless Families. *American Journal of Public Health*, 74-79, 1097-1101.

Battle, S. (1986). Social Factors in the Health of Families: A Public Health Social Work Responsibility. In G.C. St. Denis et al. (Eds.), *Proceedings, Social Factors in the Health of Families: A Public Health, Social Work Responsibility*. Division of Maternal and Child Health, Bureau of Health Care and Assistance, Department of Health and Human Services, *MCJ-000114-28*.

Butler, P.A. (1985). New Initiatives in Financing and Delivering Health Care for the Mentally Indigent: Report on a Conference, *Law Medicine and Health Care*, 13, 225-227.

Center of Budget and Policy Priorities, Analysis of Change in Food Stamp Participation (1986).

Chelimsky, E. (1982). Statement before the Sub-Committee on Human Resources in the Runaway Homeless Youth Program. U.S. House of Representatives, Committee on Education and Labor. Washington, D.C.: U.S. Government Printing Office.

Guttmacher, A. (1981). *Teenage Pregnancy: The Problem That Hasn't Gone Away*. New York: Guttmacher Institute.

Homeless Families in Massachusetts: Progress and Action. (1987). Boston: Executive Office of Human Services.

Levitan, S. (1969). Families at Risk: A Public Health Social Work Perspective. In G.C. St. Denis et al. (Eds.), *Proceedings, Families at Risk: A Public Health Social Work Perspective*. University of Pittsburgh School of Public Health, Pittsburgh, PA.

Palmer, J.L. & Sawhill, I.V. (1982). *The Reagan Record—An Urban Institute Study*, 177, Ballinger, Cambridge, MA.

Physicians Task Force on Hunger in America. (1985). *Hunger in America*. Middletown: Wesleyan University Press.

Reyes, L. & Waxman. (1986). *The Growth of Hunger, Homelessness and Poverty in America's Cities: A 25 City Survey*. U.S. Conference of Mayors.

U.S. Department of Housing and Urban Development (1984). *A Report to the Secretary on The Homeless and Emergency Shelters*. Washington, D.C.: U.S. Government Printing Office.

Adrift in the City:
A Comparative Study of Street Children
in Bogotá, Colombia, and Guatemala City

Mark Connolly

ABSTRACT. The life style of homeless children in two South American cities is reported in this chapter. The chapter describes a society within a society complete with mores, sanctions and values. The author's use of the term "street children" forces the reader to consider the dramatic and disruptive effect of poverty on children. The conclusions suggest a national policy review if the United States is to avoid a similar situation.

Throughout Latin America there are thousands of neglected children struggling to survive on the streets of all major urban areas. These youngsters can generally be seen lingering around parks and street corners, shining shoes, begging at crowded intersections, or singing for small change on city buses. After dark, they sleep huddled together on the pavement, using cardboard cartons and newspapers to make street accommodations as comfortable as possible. Frequently characterized by their uncleanliness and lawless activities, street children are thought of as pathetic waifs, despised and feared by the more affluent citizens. Recent estimates have cited some 40 million abandoned children in Latin America, and their numbers are said to be on the increase (Hoge, 1971). This phenomenon has reached alarming levels in Brazil, where more than 20 million children are growing up in the streets, and in Colombia, where the so-called *gamines* (street urchins) are a highly visible mass and a principal attraction for foreign journalists. In addition,

Mark Connolly is affiliated with CHILDHOPE in Guatemala, an international research advocacy and service organization.

Colombia's capital city, Bogotá, has an international reputation as the "abandoned child capital of the world." While an accurate census is not possible, conservative estimates of the city's street child population are between 3,000-5,000. With little support from the traditional institutions of family, school, church, or state, their efforts to survive in the streets are often seen by the public as offensive and worthy of negative social sanctions. As a result, *gamines* all over Latin America are victims of violence and repression, as their basic human needs are often misunderstood and ignored.

While known as *"chamacos,"* in Mexico, *"pibes,"* in Argentina, *"cabritos,"* in Chile, and *"botijas,"* in Uruguay, the Colombian term *gamines* is the most recognized label for vagrant Latin American street children. This phenomenon, however, is not new or limited to the region, as street boys have existed in many European and American cities. They can be also found in urban settings throughout the developing world. The situation seems to be more critical in Latin America, though, where the problem of street children stems from the glaringly unequal distribution of wealth and the social disruption caused by the rapid growth of the already crowded cities. Other factors are related to the economic and social structures of society, including external influences which condition and limit change in the urban poor environment. For example, the daily struggle to survive has become increasingly difficult in the many countries affected by the region's current economic crisis. The problem is primarily in the cities where the extreme poverty of the slums and the absence of traditional family support have led to increased abandonment of young children.

Although there are both government and private programs throughout the Americas which attempt to address what is perceived as a "street kid" problem, most are very formal and restrictive in nature, and the child tends to be regarded as either a delinquent or deviant. Children who have spent a considerable amount of time living on the streets frequently run away from such facilities in order to return to the liberty and adventure of street life. Government authorities and others use this sort of information as evidence to support the common belief that these children are uneducable delinquents, well beyond any help from society. In Colombia and Guatemala, there are several institutional programs operated by religious groups and private organizations. Some of these programs differ from government facilities in that they employ a more progressively-oriented approach to the problem of abandoned children. However, even these programs do not offer large-scale solutions for the *gamin* problem.

In general, street children can be divided into two distinct categories. The first and largest category consists of those children who spend the majority of their time active on the streets, but maintain family relations and often return home at night. A much smaller category are those who band together at night for warmth and protection while sleeping on the pavement. Such children are either truly abandoned or have chosen to leave home and live on the streets. In this article, they will be referred to as "hard-core" *gamines*, for they often bear the physical and emotional scars of a rugged street life, which has taught them to endure hostile and difficult situations.

IMAGES OF THE STREET CHILD: A REVIEW

The street child phenomenon in Latin America first received widespread attention in the early 1950s, with Luis Bunuel's famous film *Los Olvidados* (The Forgotten Ones), a memorable tale of street urchins in the outskirts of Mexico City. More recently, Hector Babenco's award-winning Brazilian film *Pixote* is perhaps the most powerful, yet realistic portrayal of the hardships and violence of life on the streets.

Most of the literature on street children has dealt exclusively with the Colombian *gamines*. Unfortunately, there have been very few comprehensive investigations or case studies that provide information about how the *gamines* live and think, particularly within their *galladas* (organized groups). Muñoz and Pachon (1980) offer one of the most complete studies available, which includes in-depth information about the hierarchical organization of the *galladas* and the realities of street life. A frequently cited study of *gamines* was done by Granados Téllez, (1974), in collaboration with the Pontificia Universidad Javeriana. While this provides a great deal of statistical information about a sample population of Bogotá street children, there is little attempt to analyze the relations between *gamines* and society. A study done by Beltrán Cortes (1969) is more of a psychological analysis of *gaminismo*, but it does not include extensive information about actual life on the streets. Finally, a fascinating autobiography of a former *gamin*, presented by Rusque-Alcaino and Bromley (1979), provides a life history of a poor Colombian, which includes a personalized view of *gaminismo* and life on the streets.

In addition to the few studies about Colombian *gamines*, other texts are useful in order to view the street child phenomenon in a broader perspective. The collection of essays presented in *Changing Childhood* (Hoyles, 1979) examines the origins, history, and political framework of childhood in different cultural settings. While a principal objective of this book is to show that children have been quite different in the past, editor Martin Hoyles argues that one unchanging element in the history of childhood is that "of all oppressed groups in society, children have perhaps the hardest task in asserting their rights to equality" (p. 16). Clearly, such is the case with the *gamines*, whose rights are extremely limited, as they are victims of severe repression and scorned by adult members of society.

An interesting topic discussed in literature by Peter Fuller (Hoyles, 1979, pp. 77-108) and Magda and John McHall (1979) is the concept of children as "miniature adults," derived from social theories which claim that childhood was actually "unknown" during many historical periods, particularly in Europe during the eighteenth and nineteenth centuries. Interestingly enough, these authors feel that childhood is suppressed in the developing world today, as children of the poor are often judged by adult standards and expected to conform to adult rules. A statement by Fuller describes this situation:

> In reality, the beggar-child, the orphan, or the offspring of the destitute poor come closer than any to being miniature adults. They cannot just wear the conventions of the adult world on the outside as costume, or false self. Whatever the cost, in terms of the denial of potentialities, distortion, or pain, they have to internalize those conventions to survive. That is why

the wizened face of the shoeblack is so often that of an old man. (p. 84)

This, of course, is a very accurate description of many street children that I encountered in Bogotá and Guatemala City. In their study of *gamines*, Muñoz and Pachon (1980) fully accept this miniature adult concept, stating that a *gamin* is simply not a child.

Finally, a number of recent publications and articles have suggested that the rapid population growth of children, under the age of fifteen, in developing countries may be creating an entire "sub-race of the deprived" (Hoge, 1983). For example, Firestone feels that as a result of the disintegration of the family structure under the pressure of poverty, children are becoming so segregated from the rest of society that they have almost become another race (Hoyles, 1979). If such is the case, *gamines* are leading this transformation, as they are a class of deprived children, due to the lack of any major institutional efforts to deal with the situation in the streets.

STUDY DESIGN

This investigation is a comparative analysis of the street child phenomenon in two different Latin American contexts. It is a descriptive study which examines the group support networks and survival modes of street urchins in Bogotá, where *gamines* abound in the streets, and in Guatemala City, where many believe that a street child problem does not even exist. The following served as research foci and assumptions:

1. The street child phenomenon in the context of urban poverty is not directly the result of externally imposed social and economic conditions. It is primarily a situational adaptation to a rapidly changing family structure in the Latin American urban environment, which mediates the larger socio-economic conditions.
2. The attitudes and values of the *gamines* distinguish them from slum children and the masses of other abandoned youngsters. Most of them have abandoned homes which they found intol-

erable and have adopted an alternative lifestyle in order to survive on the streets.
3. Although they are frequently regarded as a separate subculture, street children are just one segment of the urban street poor. In both cities, they are among the thousands of people whose work is often referred to as casual work or marginal occupations.

METHODOLOGIES AND INVESTIGATION SITES

Two distinct field experiences have provided much of the firsthand information presented in this paper. During the fall semester of 1981, I did an extensive amount of volunteer work with *gamines* in Bogotá. More recently, the summer months of 1983 were spent conducting research in Guatemala and the nearby Department of Sacatepéquez. In both cities, my approach was action-oriented, in that the studies were conducted while providing basic health care services for the street children.

Methodologies

The research techniques employed in both studies included informal interviewing and participant observation. A diary-journal was kept to record the characteristics of street life, concentrating specifically on the interaction of the street children with each other and the rest of society.

Bogotá

In Bogotá, my opportunity to study street children was greatly facilitated by becoming one of the first trained health workers for the Children of the Americas foundation. This program was founded in 1979, in an attempt to address the health care needs of the city's *gamin* population, while also providing the care and attention that is so often missing from their lives. As a healthworker, I was trained in basic first-aid and was indoctrinated into the program's "street delivery system" (Bentley & Rivo, 1982). In order to effectively minister to the needs of the street children, it was essential to become well known in some of the poorest, most violent areas of the city. Most of this work was done directly in the streets — in parks, on street corners, and in doorways. Services were provided with no questions asked and no values imposed. As a result of this approach, I was able to earn the trust and confidence of the street children, which was then maintained by being available and providing follow-up care.

In the urban areas where groups of *gamines* were concentrated, there was rarely a moment when I was not interacting with children. The basic health care services were provided informally, because *gamines* are very active and mobile during the daytime. A lot of time was spent conversing with street boys, listening to their stories, and just watching the "street action." This interaction with the *gamines* frequently attracted attention, and passersby would often stop to warn me that my young companions were dangerous and not to be trusted. Also, on a few occasions the police were suspicious of these activities, resulting in my being searched and questioned.

Throughout my stay in Colombia, a diary-journal was kept of all street work experiences. Notes were made at the end of the day, recording observations and health-related information about various "patients" and case histories of the many *gamines* encountered in different areas of the city. The children with whom I spent more time, I asked informal interview questions about their life history and living conditions. Usually, the questions were brought up during conversation and responses were not recorded in their presence. Detailed personal information was gathered from those who were my close acquaintances.

The basic research techniques were utilized in Colombia. The circumstances were different, however, in that my research in Guatemala was conducted during a shorter period and with fewer children. Furthermore, less time was spent delivering health care to street children because I also was visiting and conducting interviews at a number of public and private child care programs. A major difference between the two cities is that information regarding where *gamines* were likely to be found in Colombia had to be gathered before the investigation was fully extended out into the streets. It did not take long to discover the poorer, more dangerous neighborhoods where street children were sleeping in doorways or shining shoes.

BACKGROUND INFORMATION
AND INVESTIGATION SITES

Bogotá

The present population of Bogotá exceeds five million (Brooks, 1983) and as a result of the country's estimated urban population growth rate of 4.5%, Bogotá has become one of the fastest growing cities in Latin America (Wilkie & Harber, 1982). Furthermore, Bogotá is one of the most densely populated Latin American cities with an estimated 1799 people per square kilometer. As the population continues to grow, more *barrios clandestinos* (shantytowns) are appearing on the outskirts of the city. Most of the street children either come from these settlements or the low-income neighborhoods located in the central city.

Although Colombia is currently regarded as a politically stable and democratic country, there has been a great deal of political and social upheaval in recent history. Particularly during the 1930s and 1940s, there was a tremendous struggle between the two major political parties which set the stage for a long period of political violence. Between 1948 and 1957, a bloody civil war known as *La Violencia* drove many rural families into the cities and left some 300,000 people dead in the countryside (Brooks, 1983). This tremendous split between the Liberals and the Conservatives was resolved in 1957 and a relatively stable, centralized government has been maintained up to the present.

While violent social disorder no longer exists in the rural areas of Colombia, exceedingly high crime rates have made many of the larger cities quite dangerous. Almost every traveller or tourist that has been to this city has stories to tell about being robbed or witnessing a crime in the streets. Unfortunately, it is in this context that the subject of *gamines* is frequently mentioned, for they are ever-present, roaming the dangerous streets of the city.

Most of the children that I worked with were hardcore *gamines*, meaning that they lived, ate, and slept on the streets. They were concentrated in the central area of the city, very near the bus terminals and the downtown business district. Although travelling around the city was not uncommon, most of their daily activities took place within a three-block radius of the *Parque de los Már-tires*, a small plaza which is a notorious gathering place for thieves, prostitutes, drug dealers, and *gamines*. Nearby neighborhoods such as *El Cartucho*, *Los Escombros*, and *La Once* are also considered very dangerous, because they are more inconspicuous havens for these people. This general area was commonly referred to as *la selva* (the jungle). Two other significant locations for the *gamines* are the *Plaza España* and *La Rebeca* fountain. The first site is a market for second-hand goods and used clothing, located near a garbage dump and the bus terminals. *Gamines* are regular customers at the plaza, often purchasing clothing and shoes, or selling stolen items to the vendors. *La Rebeca* on the other hand, is a popular bathing spot for *gamines*, located across from the luxurious Tequendama hotel. Recently, their skinny-dipping in this public fountain has attracted a great deal of publicity, and police officers are now under orders to chase them out.

Guatemala City

Guatemala is the most populous country in Central America with an estimated 7.9 million people (Population Reference Bureau, 1983). Also, it is one of the few Latin American countries that has a predominantly Indian population. For the most part, Guatemala is an agricultural nation that depends heavily on the exportation of coffee, cotton, bananas, and sugar for revenue to support the impoverished economy. The industrial sector is growing steadily, exporting primarily to other countries in the region (Brooks, 1983). An estimated thirty-seven percent of the population lives in urban areas, yet aside from the capital there is no other city with a population exceeding 100,000. The urban growth rate for this country is cited as 2.1% (Wilkie & Haber, 1982), much of which is experienced in Guatemala City, which has a population of about 1,180,000 (Brooks, 1983). Located on a plateau 1,500 meters above sea level, Guatemala City enjoys a very temperate climate and only light rainfall. The city is very large and spread out with a population density of 530.5 per square kilometer (Wilkie & Haber, 1982). There are over twenty metropolitan *zonas* (zones), ranging from the central *Zona 1* to the unnumbered shantytowns along the outskirts of the city.

Aside from the extensive destruction and damage caused by a 1976 earthquake which left 23,000 dead, Guatemala has also been racked by recent political violence. In some cases, the civil violence has caused rural families to relocate in cities and towns. Others have simply fled their villages and headed for refugee camps located along the Mexican frontier.

As could be expected, an overall result of this political instability is that Guatemala's orphaned and abandoned child population is noticeably on the increase. While most of these children are dealt with in the areas of conflict, many are now being referred to institutional programs in the capital city and the surrounding area. Although it has yet to be determined whether these young victims of the civil strife have significantly altered the city's street child population, a continued flow of these abandonees would increase the likelihood of more children showing up in the streets in the near future.

While many abandoned children can be found in government facilities and private programs, the children that are never heard about are the ones who make it on their own, those who do not fall into the hands of the exploiters, social agencies, or the police. In Guatemala City, countless youngsters can be seen during the day, lingering around the parks and streetcorners of virtually every urban zone. However, it is the hardcore *gamines* who roam the busy streets of Zone 1 at night, or sleep under buses at the *Terminal*. Street children do not abound in this city and a number of days were spent walking around the metropolitan ares before a *gallada* was encountered. These boys were between the ages of 8 and 16, and formed a loosely structured group that gathered near the *Plaza Barrios* in Zone 1. Their particular territory is between *Calles 15-18* and *Avenidas 7-11*. Many of them shine shoes near the plaza or at the few bus stations nearby. While this area is relatively safe during the day, it is rather dangerous after dark, as all-night taverns are the focal point of illicit activities which include prostitution and drug sales. The street boys are very visible characters in this scenario, lying huddled together on the sidewalks or curled up in doorways.

THE LIFE CYCLE OF A GAMIN

Although it is commonly believed that many street children were orphaned or physically abandoned at an early age, such children actually constitute the smallest category of *gamines*. For most street urchins, much of childhood is spent as a member of a low-income family, living in a poor urban area. The traditional family structure is often disrupted and a variety of family situations are produced. Some of the more common arrangements include combined families (where two separated parents bring their children into a new family grouping); female-headed households; legal marriages; and consensual unions. In any case, the family structure is substantially weakened by the pressures of survival, which require all but the youngest children to help support the family.

As children of the urban poor in Latin America grow older, girls are more needed within the family, as they are expected to perform household chores and care for younger siblings. Young males, on the other hand, are often less subject to adult controls and tend to become more aggressive and independent (McHale, 1979). As early as six or seven years of age, male children begin spending more time away from the household, wandering around or playing with other neighborhood children. At this *"pre-gamin"* stage, the child becomes familiar with street life and the first few excursions through downtown streets reveal a hazardous but completely new world. The initial enticement to life in the streets usually stems from the child's envy of the adventurous and apparently carefree lifestyle of the *gamines*. Particularly in Colombia, neighborhood adolescents with "street experience" are also very influential characters, as they talk of easily earning money by begging or stealing. This situation is well exemplified by a former *gamin's* statement that "I saw other petty thieves who were big—sixteen-years-old and twelve-years-old—and of course I wanted to do the same as them" (Rusque-Alcaino & Bromley, 1979).

As the child becomes increasingly interested in *gaminismo*, more time is spent on the streets observing boys his own age earning money and spending it on whatever they desire. Yet, as the child gradually breaks away from the home environment, a situation of conflict arises because the young individual is expected to contribute to the family income. Furthermore, parents usually strongly disapprove of their child roaming the streets with "delinquents." As a result, the rising tension often leads to physical abuse and punishment on a regular basis. Finally, when the situation becomes unbearable, the child will abandon the household, opting for life on the streets.

Family Situations and Living Conditions

In order to illustrate some of the more unstable family situations and living conditions, I will describe two households which had been abandoned by discontented young males. In one *colonia* (marginal neighborhood) in Guatemala City, a family of seven lived in a shack that had rough wooden planks for walls, a roof of corrugated metal, and a dirt floor. According to the middle-age mother, her husband is an alcoholic and strikes the children when he is drunk. Their income is equivalent to approximately $50.00 a month. It comes mostly from the father's job of washing and guarding automobiles in the downtown district. The mother occasionally earns money by washing clothes, but most of her time is spent preparing meals and keeping the house clean. This family spends about $2.00 each day on food supplies, which are predominantly rice, cornmeal, and black beans. Finally, the rent for their property is equal to $6.00 per month. They have been in debt to the landowner for the past three years.

As far as the children are concerned, all of them are illiterate even though a public school is located within one-hundred yards of their home. None of them have attended classes because they are needed to perform household chores and take care of each other. Furthermore, they are all undernourished and exposed to a number of health risks. Their playground is an area of open sewers and garbage dumps, in which disease is an ever-constant threat. In regard to their future, the mother admits that she is incapable of providing proper attention and she only hopes that God will in some way make life better for her children. Over the past two years, two of her young sons have left home, after violent arguments with their father. For them, life in the streets may in fact be better than what is offered by the home environment, as neither child has returned.

In visiting another household, I met an attractive, twenty-nine year old woman, who lives alone with her five children. Their house is made of wood, with a dirt floor, and consists of a bedroom, a kitchen, and a latrine. Although there is no running water, they do have electricity, but it is not included in the monthly rent of about $50.00. Both mother and children are illiterate and no attempts have been made to enroll any of the children in school. The oldest daughter is fourteen years old and she is responsible for keeping the house clean and making sure that her brothers and sisters are fed. The younger ones spend most of the day at their neighbor's house, where a close friend takes care of them. Three of the children are from the mother's marriage, but since her husband left, she has had two others by different men. One of the fathers does provide financial support for his child, but the mother must work day and night in order to adequately support the rest of the family. While part of her income comes from washing clothes and domestic work, her involvement in prostitution is an important economic supplement, especially in times of hardship.

As far as the future of her children is concerned, this woman openly admits that she feels incompetent to raise them properly. She would like to turn the children over to government homes or other social agencies, simply because she does not want to be responsible for them. On the other hand, she does care for them and was very concerned about her eleven-year-old son, who had been hanging around a "bad neighborhood" and often did not come home at night. However, she did not know how to improve their living conditions or possibly convince her son to remain with the family.

Survival on the Streets

Once the child has left home and decided to live on the streets, he usually comes in contact with other street boys, in the context of a *gallada*. For street urchins between the ages of eight and sixteen, the *gallada* is a vital social structure for both individual and collective survival on the streets. It not only protects the members against the threat of crime and exploitation, but it also serves to meet their emotional and physical needs. Although there are varying degrees of organization amongst these groups, each individual member has a way of interaction which remains stable and fixed through continual group activity. For example, once becoming a member of a *gallada*, the young male will spend much time playing with new friends, going to the movies with them, and most importantly, he will learn to survive on the streets. While most of the *gallada*'s daytime activities are concerned with foraging for survival, at night, *gamines* gather together to form a *camada*, which is a smaller group of boys who sleep in a common area for warmth and protection.

In Bogotá, there are essentially two types of *galladas*: one for younger *gamines* between the ages of eight and eleven, and another for older boys and adolescents. In general, the younger children form loosely organized groups, which are primarily concerned with satisfying basic survival needs. For the most part, these youngsters, known as *"chinches"* (bedbugs), simply beg for food and money, and are not involved with illegal activities. They are also frequently considered to be cute or comical characters, and as a result have little difficulty obtaining enough money to take care of themselves.

The *galladas* comprised of older boys are renowned and feared in Colombia because they are often regarded as gangs of young thieves. These *galladas* are usually highly structured groups, in which there is a clear division of work, a rigid system of sanctions, and a well-defined method of dividing their earnings. In short, each member knows exactly what his role is within the group. For example, in the *Parque de los Mártires* area, one encounters *gamines* dedicated specifically to pocket picking, robbing watches, begging for food, or selling stolen objects. Another unique characteristic of these *galladas* is that a clear leadership hierarchy exists, which is dominated by older boys. In general, the group leaders are skilled fighters, not easily intimidated, and are well connected with adult criminals and other street people. These leaders coordinate the activities of the group, which include the selection of territory and distribution of their collective earnings among group members.

In Guatemala City the situation is quite different in that the highly structured *gallada* is virtually non-existent and there does not appear to be separate groupings of younger children. Overall, membership in *galladas* is rather loose and informal, including both hardcore *gamines* and younger boys who are only on the street during the day. The street boys encountered in the *Plaza Barrios* area, however, did interact with a high level of frequency and their activities followed a relatively fixed pattern. For the most part, each of them owned a shine box and obtained some of his income from shining shoes. Interestingly enough, they put their supplies away after one or two shines, in order to concentrate on other activities. Begging for leftover food at restaurants was a common practice, as was petty thievery. In Guatemala City, however, the participation in hard crime appears to be on a much less serious scale than in Bogotá. Finally, leadership roles were not well-defined in these *galladas*, but older boys were the most respected and group activities centered around them.

In Guatemala City and Bogotá, income opportunities for *gamines* range from begging or shining shoes, to petty thievery and violent crime. On the whole, survival modes and lifestyle often depend upon the preferred activities of the *gallada* in their respective environment. In order to compare life on the streets in these two cities, I have chosen to examine the health concerns of *gamines*, as indicators of their struggle to survive and the overall situation in the streets.

As could be expected, the violent streets of Bogotá make life exceedingly hazardous for the street children. Knife and gunshot wounds are commonplace and street accidents resulting in the loss of a limb or an eye are routine. The most common ailments include infected lacerations, burns, contusions, headlice, fleas, and sores of all description. As victims of severe repression and negative social sanctions, *gamines* have little access to health care because clinics, health centers, and even emergency wards refuse them treatment. Furthermore, the *gamin* learns at an early age to shun such facilities because he often faces questioning by police or other officials, who assume that a wounded *gamin* is criminally responsible for his own injury. In fact, it is a fairly common occurrence that following an interrogation, the child is sent to jail untreated.

While street boys in Guatemala City experience a similar inaccessibility to most health care facilities, they rarely have to fear police questioning in an emergency situation. On the whole, these *gamines* are not as exposed to major health risks and street violence. While a few of them displayed small scars or handicaps from street accidents, nothing compared to the wounds and scars observed daily on virtually every Bogotá *gamin*. As a result, the medical attention which they needed involved treating minor lacerations, burns, and bruises. As in Colombia, there were also widespread occurrences of scabies, fleas, headlice, and tineapedis (foot fungus). Finally, in both cities the street environment is not very conducive to maintaining proper hygiene, so that the only real preventive measures for *gamines* are alertness and common sense.

The problem of drug use is also a health-related concern which has a major impact on street survival. While hard drugs are virtually unknown among *gamines*, a variety of intoxicants and narcotics are used to provide relief from the pain of cold and hunger. In both locations, the most common and injurious form of "getting high" is the sniffing of glue or gasoline fumes. These substances are very accessible on the street and a "high" can be maintained all day, with a thirty-cent bottle of shoe cement. The heavy users are easily recognized by their ragged clothing, soiled faces, and glazed eyes, and the effects of brain damage are observable among long-time users. In Bogotá, *gamines* also favor marijuana and *bazuka*, which is a smoking mix of tobacco and cocaine. These drugs are less available and more expensive in Guatemala, where drinking is a more common practice amongst the street boys.

To summarize the principal aspects of the street child phenomenon, it should be emphasized that most *gamines* have fled mistreatment and abuse suffered at home in favor of the unwelcoming streets of the city. Having looked at some of the poorer living conditions in Guatemala City shantytowns, leaving home may very well be a positive, adaptive move towards improved physical and psychological health. In any case, "making it" on the streets almost always hinges upon acceptance into a *gallada*. As a member of such a group, be it loosely organized or highly structured, the street child is relatively protected from exploitation and becomes familiar with the low-status or illegal street occupations which are income opportunities for *gamines*.

For those who decide to "go straight," available income opportunities include street vending or other low-paying employment in restaurants, bars, and small shops. In Bogotá and Guatemala City, work may also take the form of "ragpicking," which entails pulling a wooden cart through the streets, seeking out anything collectable: cloth, cardboard, glass, plastic, or wood. Other forms of work within the service sector include guarding parked cars, selling lottery tickets, or shining shoes. As members of the urban poor, they must work hard to earn a meager living to support themselves and their households. The prevailing socio-economic structure, however, severely limits upward mobility, so that there are few chances of ever escaping their situation of poverty.

Finally, it should be noted that not all *gamines* survive the hostile and difficult conditions of life on the streets. A truly abandoned child, for example, is often the one that the family was least able to care for, perhaps because he suffers from some neurological disorder or physical impairment. Such children are least equipped to face life in the streets, but there are few care facilities that can offer an alternative. There is no doubt that many simply perish. Furthermore, urban violence and street fights, especially in Bogotá, make death "the *gamin*'s constant street companion" (Bentley & Rivo, 1982). In many cases, knife and gunshot wounds are the cause of death, while tragic street accidents claim others. Thus, while most *gamines* have the ability and are fortunate enough to survive, their lifestyle is inherently dangerous and the street claims many young victims.

CONCLUSION

Gaminismo represents a situational adaptation to a changing family structure in urban environments throughout Latin America. The two low-income households in Guatemala City shantytowns are illustrative of such family situations which were unbearable for some children. In the first case, the family lived under extreme conditions of poverty and the children were not adequately cared for or supported. While the father did earn a minimal income by washing and guarding automobiles, the children also had to share responsibility for the sustenance of the family. The situation was exacerbated by the fact that the father had a serious drinking problem and frequently abused the children. As a result of the lack of protection and emotional security within this family structure, two of the boys fled the mistreatment in favor of life on the streets.

The woman living alone with her five children also represents a situation that differs from the traditional nuclear family structure. While the mother works exceptionally hard to support the family, the children are needed to perform household chores and take care of each other. As a result of having only one parent at home, these children do not receive sufficient attention to basic childhood necessities. Furthermore, it is also evident in this case that such circumstances have weakened the family structure and led the oldest son to abandon the household. In both Colombia and Guatemala, most *gamines* come from such lower class backgrounds and their increasing numbers is a consequence of the socio-economic deprivation which disrupts families and often forces children into the streets in order to survive.

Gamines differ from other poor, disadvantaged children in that they have adopted an alternative lifestyle, independent of the basic nuclear family. In both Guatemala City and Bogotá, it is evident that the *gallada* replaces the family as the principal socializing unit for street children, serving to protect them and meet their emotional needs. On the whole, these groups are relatively well organized and demonstrate very efficient systems of taking care of themselves. The *galladas* of the *Parque de los Mártires* (Bogotá) and the *Plaza Barrios* (Guatemala City), for example, are self-sufficient, as they provide their own food, shelter, and clothing. In fact, their problem is not a lack of organization, but a failure of their own social organization to mesh with the structure of society around it.

Although street life is often considered to be a vicious struggle to survive under oppressive conditions of poverty, living conditions on the street are often better than those at home. Aside from the relative abundance of food, other advantages of street life include an unrestricted environment, an opportunity to earn money, and participation in exciting and adventurous activities. In order to get by, however, street children must take advantage of any opportunity that comes along and adopt those values and patterns of behavior that will help them survive.

The activities of *gamines* in both cities confirm that street children constitute a significant segment of the lower working class in the urban centers of Latin America. Many work in non-waged or extremely low-waged jobs, such as begging or shining shoes, the line between legal and illegal activities is not very clear, and in order to remain on the streets one must be agile enough to cross back and forth across the line. In either situation, be it a legal or illegal income opportunity, street children are clearly earning a living and are therefore part of the working population.

One final conclusion that can be drawn is that the number of street children in Bogotá and Guatemala City can be expected to increase as continuing population growth intensifies pressure on the physical infrastructure of urban areas. Furthermore, as long as governments fail to respond to human need by ignoring the socio-economic causes of marginality, more children will be forced to roam the streets.

REFERENCES

Ardila, R. (1981). Que paso con los gamines? *El Tiempo*, 9 de Noviembre, Bogotá.

Beltrán, C. & Luis, M. (1969). *Temas Colombianos: La metamorfosis del Chino de la calle*. Bogotá: Editextos Ltda., 1-65.

Bentley, W. (1981). Images on the Death of a Gamin, *Hola*, October, 9.

Bentley, W. & Marc, R. (1982). *Meeting Health Needs of Street Children on Their Turf: Their Terms*. Unpublished paper delivered at the American Public Health Association and American College of Preventive Medicine combined sessions, Montreal, November 16.

Bromley, R. & Chris, G. (Ed.) (1979). *Casual Work and Poverty in Third World Cities*. New York: John Wiley and Sons.

Brooks, J. (Ed.) (1983). *The 1983 South American Handbook: Traveller's Guide to Latin America and the Caribbean*. Bath, England: Trade and Travel Publications.

DeNicolo, J., Irenarcco Ardila E., Camilo Castrellon P., & German, M. (1981). *Musaranas*. Bogotá: Industria Continental Grafica.

Felsman, K. (1981). Street Urchins of Colombia, *Natural History*, April, 40-49.

Feracuti, F. (1975). *Delinquents and Non-Delinquents in the Puerto Rican Slum Culture*. Columbus, Ohio: The Ohio State University.

Figueroa Vides, S. (1967). El Adolescente Guatemalteco Frente al Derecho Penal. Guatemala: Universidad de San Carlos de Guatemala.

Goffman, E. (1962). *Asylums*. Chicago: Aldine Publishing.

148   *Homeless Children: The Watchers and the Waiters*

Goffman, E. (1967). *Interaction Ritual: Essays on Face-to-Face Behavior*. New York: Anchor Books Doubleday and Company, Inc.

Goffman, E. (1974). *Frame Analysis: An Essay on the Organization of Experience*. New York: Harper and Row Publishers.

Higgins, S.J. (1979). *Shoeshines, Street Life, and Survival: A Study of the Gamines in Quito, Ecuador*. M.A. thesis, University of Texas, Austin.

Hoge, W. (1983). For Every One We Reach There are 1,000 We Don't Touch, *New York Times*, September 11, 8E.

Hoyles, M. (Ed.) (1979). *Changing Childhood*. London: Writers and Readers Publishing Cooperative.

La Fuente, E.E. (1979). *Integractión Familiar y Adaptación Psicosocial Estudio en un Grupo de Adolescentes Guatemaltecas*. Guatemala: Universidad de San Carlos de Guatemala.

Leacock, E.B. (Ed.) (1971). *The Culture of Poverty: A Critique*. New York: Basic Books.

Lewis, O. (1959). *Five Families: Mexican Case Studies in the Culture of Poverty*. New York: Basic Books.

Lewis, O. (1966). *La Vida: A Puerto Rican Family in the Culture of Poverty – San Juan and New York*. New York: Random House.

Liebow, E. (1967). *Tally's Corner: A Study of Negro Streetcorner Men*. Boston: Little, Brown.

McHale, M.C. & McHale, J. (1979). World of Children, *Population Bulletin*, 33 (6). Washington, D.C.: Population Reference Bureau.

Mitchell, J.C. (Ed.) (1969). The Concept and Uses of Social Networks, 1-50 in James Clyde Mitchell (Ed.), *Social Networks in Urban Situations*. Manchester: Manchester University Publishing.

Muñoz, V.C. & Pachon, X.C. (1980). *Gamines Testimonios*. Bogotá: Carlos Valencia Editores.

Perlman, J.E. (1976). *The Myth of Marginality: Urban Poverty and Politics in Rio De Janeiro*. Berkeley: University of California Press.

Population Reference Bureau. (1982a). *1982 World's Children Data Sheet*. Washington, D.C.: Population Reference Bureau.

Population Reference Bureau. (1982b). *Urban Growth in Latin America*. Washington, D.C.: Population Reference Bureau.

Population Reference Bureau. (1983). *1983 World's Data Sheet*. Washington, D.C.: Population Reference Bureau.

Riis, J.A. (1957). *How the Other Half Lives*. New York: Hill and Wang.

Roberts, B.R. (1973). *Organizing Strangers: Poor Families in Guatemala City*. Austin: University of Texas.

Roberts, B.R. (1978). *Cities of Peasants: The Political Economy of Urbanization in the Third World*. Beverly Hills: Sage Publication.

Roberts, B.R. & Lowder, S. (1970). *Urban Population Growth and Migration in Latin America: Two Case Studies by Bryan Roberts and Stella Lowder*. Liverpool: University of Liverpool.

Rusque-Alcaino, J. & Bromley, R. (1979). The Bottle Buyer: An Occupational

Autobiography, 185-214 in Ray Bromley and Chris Gerry (Eds.), *Casual Work and Poverty in Third World Cities*. New York: John Wiley and Sons.

Safa, H.I. (1971). Puerto Rican Adaptations to the Urban Milieu, 153-190 in Peter Orleans and William Russell Ellis, Jr. (Eds.), *Race, Change and Urban Society*. Beverly Hills: Sage Publications.

Sanjek, R. (1978). A Network Method and Its Uses in Urban Ethnography, *Human Organization*, 37 (3), 257-268.

Tellez, G. & Marcos, F. (1974). *Gamines*. Bogotá: Ediciones Tercer Mundo.

Valentine, C. (1968). *Culture and Poverty: Critique and Counter Proposals*. Chicago: University of Chicago Press.

Ward, C. (1978). *The Child in the City*. New York: Pantheon Books.

Whyte, W.F. (1943). *Street Corner Society: The Social Structure of an Italian Slum*. Chicago: University of Chicago Press.

Wilkie, J.W. & Haber, S. (Eds.) (1982). *Statistical Abstract of Latin America*, 21. Los Angeles: UCLA Latin American Center Publications, University of California.

Wilkie, J.W. & Haber, S. (Eds.) (1983). *Statistical Abstract of Latin America*, 22. Los Angeles: UCLA Latin American Center Publications, University of California.

Index